VIEW FROM THE BED

✥

VIEW FROM THE BEDSIDE

WISING UP ANTHOLOGIES

www.universaltable.org

ILLNESS & GRACE, TERROR & TRANSFORMATION
2007

FAMILIES: THE FRONTLINE OF PLURALISM
2008

LOVE AFTER 70
2008

DOUBLE LIVES, REINVENTION & THOSE WE LEAVE BEHIND
2009

VIEW FROM THE BED

VIEW FROM THE BEDSIDE

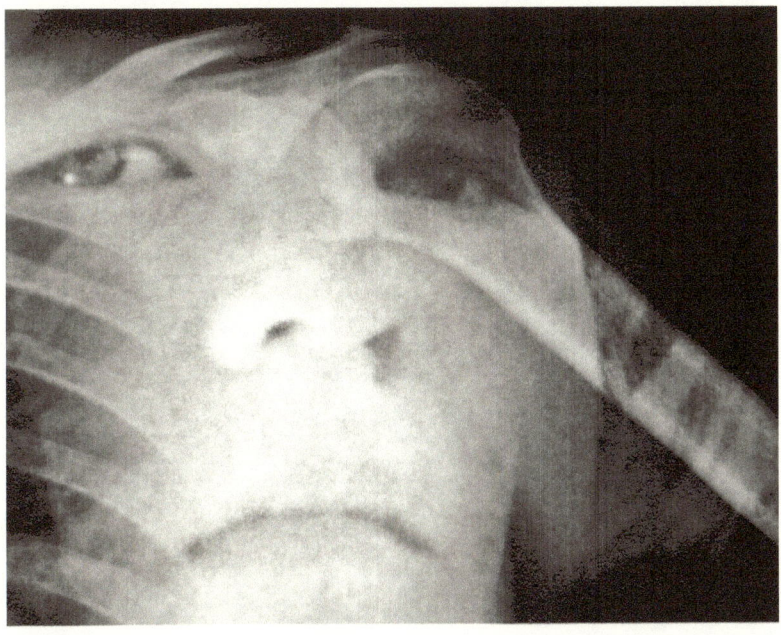

Heather Tosteson, Phyllis A. Langton, Charles D. Brockett
Editors

Wising Up Press
Decatur, Georgia

Wising Up Press
P.O. Box 2122
Decatur, GA 30031-2122
www.universaltable.org

Catalogue-in-Publication data is on file with the Library of Congress.
LCCN: 2010933327
Wising Up ISBN-13: 978-0-9827262-1-1

TABLE OF CONTENTS

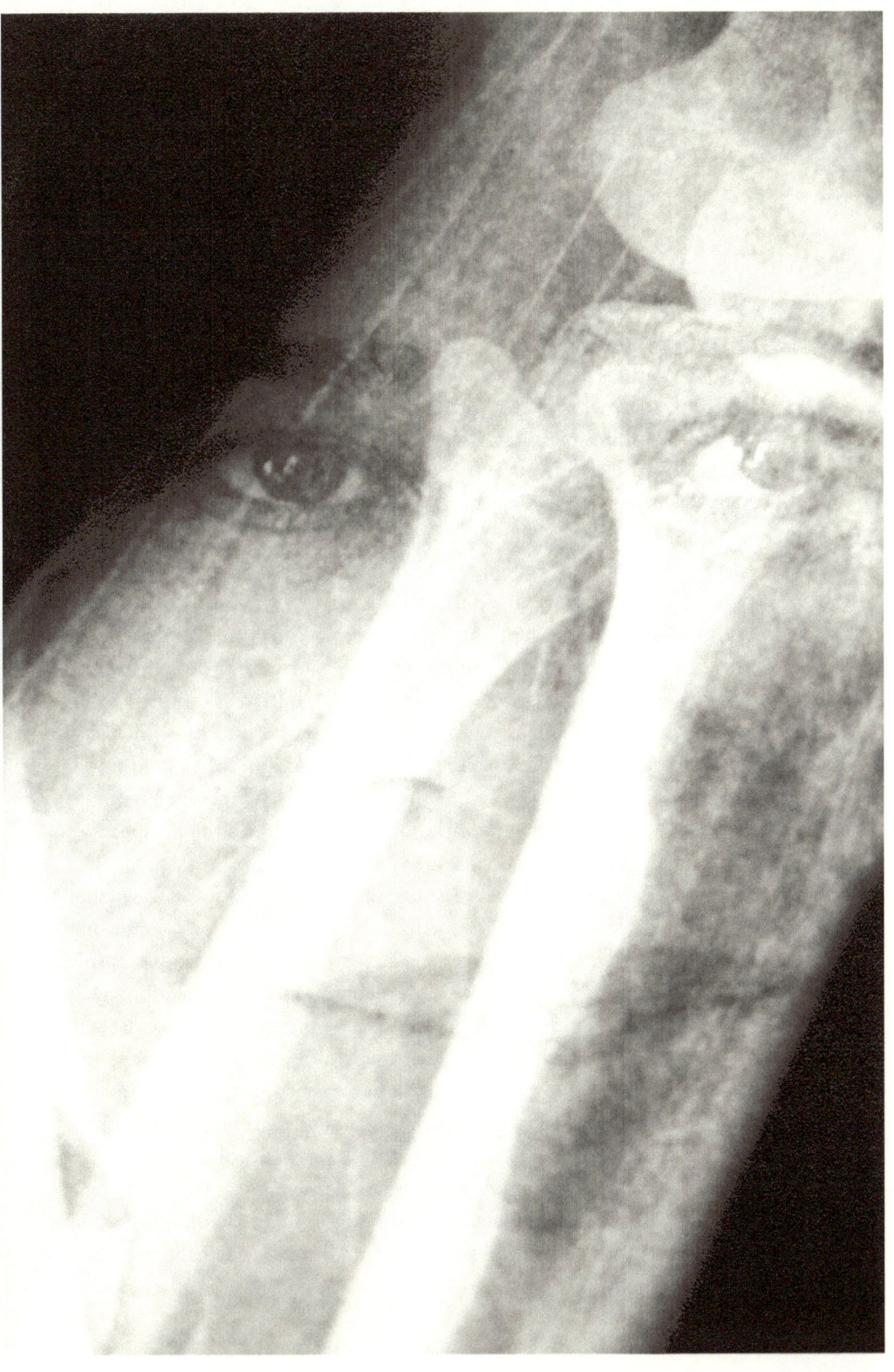

HEATHER TOSTESON

HOLDING THE WHOLE:
VIEW FROM THE BED & VIEW FROM THE BEDSIDE

I think my own interest in the different and often dissonant views from bed and bedside is over-determined. It's hard to select the most potent contributors. They derive from various personal experiences in the bed and at the bedside, often as a loving observer. What concerns me most is the experience of lost opportunity, cross-purposes, needless pain.

Much of my professional life I worked with physicians and scientists, first as a writer helping them express their thoughts clearly, then as an editor of science journals moderating their conversations with each other, and finally as a communications specialist developing training courses and doing research on professional identity formation and the role of narrative in building social trust between professionals and the public. As an editor and publisher that interest in how people explore meaning in the face of illness has continued, beginning with our first Wising Up Anthology, *Illness & Meaning; Terror & Transformation*, and now with this anthology that combines the perspectives of doctors, nurses, therapists and patients.

But my own interest has very personal roots as well and, when I think about it, may have preceded me into this world. I was born, somewhat inconveniently, in the middle of my mother's second year at Columbia University College of Physicians and Surgeons. Born on Election Day, I interfered with my mother's ability to vote—something she wrote the election board to protest when they said that childbirth did not make her eligible for an absentee ballot. My actual birth may also, from hints she later gave me, have been a source of greater personal challenge because members of her predominantly male class felt they could come and observe the birth of a vigorous and unplanned child that she was desperately searching for the energy to absorb into her life plans. I think sadly now of that combination of emotional ambivalence and physical exposure, how trapped she was then between bed and bedside.

My sisters, as children, had serious illnesses—congenital heart defect and septic kidney—but in general the attitude toward our health was dispassionate and robust. My mother didn't pander to hypochondria, brusquely offering to write a parental excuse from school if we would just stop our hypocritical coughing. She was very kind to us when we were truly felled by cold or flu, bringing us soup and sympathy. On the other hand, when in genuine duress my body tried to communicate with her through illness, it went deafeningly unheard. Instead of my mother seeing my skin disease as a sign of unusual stress, she (a dermatology resident at the time) saw its unilateral distribution as a medical oddity and proudly took me to various medical meetings as a live dermatological specimen. She was oblivious to the discomfort I felt when strange men pulled my skirt up higher and higher to see more of my lesion, which I later came to understand as an expression of my existential rebellion against earlier molestation.

For years, every time I saw a physician, I would leave, condition identified, prescription in hand, with the most profound and seemingly unmotivated feelings of despair—as if the real source of my dis-ease were, forever, undiagnosed. It's a look that I've seen on the faces of patients when busy physicians race briskly from their hospital beds leaving them to puzzle through the world-reversing implications of their diagnosis.

Like anyone, when I start thinking about my own experiences with doctors and the healthcare system, I experience a meteor shower of associations: How the nurses in the pediatric ICU watched, mesmerized, as my brother-in-law spoke to his three-year-old son in a language they didn't understand but whose tone soothed them as deeply as it did my nephew. "What is he saying?" they asked. "He's just telling him exactly what happened today, what is going to happen tomorrow," I answered. I can remember a few years later, after a less successful operation that left the surgeons sullen, reluctant to visit, telling my sister and brother-in-law, "Take your son home. They can't teach you how to live well with this." And, some years after that, parsing responsibilities with my sister so that I could question a cardiologist eager to catheterize my nephew about the risks of the procedure, that meager 60% success rate, while she listened and wept and understood exactly what it might mean for her child and herself if she made the wrong choice. I can remember my aging, Parkinson's-bent father, also a physician by training, also weeping as he pointed to a rough hand-drawn diagram of his grandson's heart, its lethally narrowing valves: "It's just a pump, a goddamn pump."

I see the expression on my husband's face when a urologist, staring at my MRI scan, casually mentioned that 90% of tumors found in kidneys are cancerous. We were meeting with him at my husband's insistence to review the results of the tests before the doctor went on a two-week white-water rafting vacation in Colorado. "No, this can't wait," my usually mild-mannered husband had told the nurse, using his own full title. "Tell him I am sure he will be able to find ten minutes in his very busy day *because it is the right thing to do.*" It had been a question of civic responsibility. "It is bad *practice*," my husband had said. And it was up to us, as enlightened consumers, to create a world we wanted to be part of.

"I insisted he fit us in because he was so inconsiderate," my husband said in the car. "I had no idea what he was sitting on. How would he feel if another doctor did that to his wife." He fumed all the way home. I was the one who, bemused, was treating this as a communications case study, noting how my facile use of medical language (and familiarity with the ominous literature) had calmed the doctor who steadfastly refused to meet my husband's gaze or shake his hand. It was easier for me to be detached—for I had already managed to receive duplicates of my scans and the radiologist's report (which was reassuring, I had a benign angiomyolipoma, not cancer) before the urologist had himself and without his knowledge. His callous behavior, predicated on a belief he was our sole source of information, may have had reasons, but really no excuse.

The list goes on, of course. The hospital clerk and gastroenterologist who before giving me a complete GI series asked me to fill out a questionnaire on sexual assault, but when queried about what use they intended to make of this information, shrugged. Standard procedure. "You ask for that information before a surgical procedure, arbitrarily activating those memories, without any plan to address them?" I asked a member of the hospital's ethics board amazed. Their intentions, of course, I never questioned—just the consequences of their social tone-deafness.

And there are, of course, powerful images on the other side: The chief resident who held my hand during childbirth. The tall white-haired patrician surgeon who visited regularly with my nephew and his family whatever the outcome. The oncologist at the University of Pennsylvania I once shadowed through a typical day who said quietly, "I like this specialty. There is always something, however small, I can do to make my patient more comfortable." The wonderful family medicine practitioner I have now who, when I asked about nutrition and inflammation said that her own knowledge was limited and then pulled out her phone and dialed her mother, who had thoroughly researched alternative treatments for her fibromyalgia, and handed the phone to me so we could consult directly.

But this question of missed opportunities, of cross-purposes, has a keen and present edge to it too, one that brings us directly to the purpose of this anthology.

In my early fifties I went through several years of profound depression. I understood it to be a response to life pressures, ones that felt close to insuperable, and also the answer to a prayer—a profound need to know myself fully before I died. I was clear that I wanted to get through this anguishing time without drugs. I had seen my own mother hospitalized, given electric shock, drugged stuporous with Miltown, which she replaced soon enough with equally sedating doses of gin. As a young feminist, I felt actions, decisive actions like divorce, would have served her better. But I also knew that wasn't the answer to the challenges I faced. I needed to see my own depression as a faith journey, one that had inner coherence, a gracious purpose, if, as yet, no clear path. My husband and spiritual director were both brave enough to keep faith with me, but there was a moment early on when, with a caution I agreed with, I went at my spiritual director's suggestion to see a psychiatrist about whether drugs might be advisable.

I can remember where I was sitting—on a couch slightly lower than his office chair that he had pulled around from his desk. There was dark leather everywhere, tall bookcases, a few token pieces of art. I looked over his shoulder at his desk, his computer. I knew my spiritual director thought highly of him, but I can still remember how I understood almost immediately that it wasn't just a mistake, it was a near disaster to come and see him. It had to do with the structure of the interview itself. From his point of view it made perfect sense. He wanted to sound the depths of my despair. He wanted to know if I was a danger to myself or to others. He didn't want to know the light in me, only the dark. He wanted to know about every trauma in my life. He didn't want to know how I had resolved them, grown from them, integrated them. He *didn't* want to know my strengths, the powerful mystery of my resilience. Every time I tried to include this, he shook his head, rattled his paper impatiently. That box was already checked.

In my memory there was a point in the interview when something in me went mute in self-defense. I stopped trying to explain myself, share my story. When he looked up from his checklist, I just shrugged, rose, thanked him for his time, paid him on the spot. All I wanted to do was get out of that room, get away from someone who intended no harm but whose gaze was annihilating.

I haven't thought of that moment in many years, but it comes back to me as I read, cover to cover and back to back, various memoirs of illness. I remember how time slowed, how some part of me just stepped back refusing to help this thin, humorless, well-intentioned, unimaginative man rip away one more scab on my psyche. And all the time I was keenly aware he meant no harm—*and* that he was truly dangerous to me and my fraying life wish. In his urge to treat, he was gutting my life of meaning, stripping me of all agency. *Innocently.*

Reviewing Rita Charon's *Narrative in Medicine* yesterday in preparation for writing this introduction, I came to a shocked standstill before the word *pathographies*, which she used a little hesitantly as a description of memoirs of illness. When I read it, I had a similar sensation to what I had a little later when I recalled this episode with the psychiatrist. *Pathography*, I thought, sounding the word out. *Pathological. Pathetic.* My life as a disease. That poor man who didn't know me from Eve was listening loyally for my *pathography* while I was, in one of the darkest periods of my life, living the namelessness that was mine alone to live as a blessing story, one that was, it was true, leading me deep into a dark and seemingly endless wood.

There is a movement now to study the role of narrative in medicine, to apply the techniques of literary analysis to the stories patients tell, to train physicians to listen for story, which I too think is crucial. But even more crucial is what kind of story we are listening for—and whether it bears any relation at all to the one that, whatever the encroaching circumstances, blesses our continuous dying into life and living into death. *That* one, the one we can't imagine ourselves without, the one we can't imagine for ourselves at all unless we are securely held in someone's imagination, some one person more than ourselves. That story does not know itself as a *pathography* or its protagonist as *pathographer* even if its catalyst is illness.

I think of the memoir *Sick Girl* and Amy Silverstein's inner response when her doctor, seventeen years into her heart transplant, asks in response to her despair and expressed doubts about the value of going on, "What gives your life meaning?" She realizes that her focus has simply been on survival, and knows that is not enough. She turns to writing and discovers there that more spacious story inside which she is truly free to share her reality, eloquent, biting, undistorted, with those whose lives, too, have been consumed by their desire for her survival. For to know ourselves to be held whole in someone else's imagination is to begin to hold their reality as tenderly and faithfully in our own. The slightest glimpse, actually, will do. That's really all we are asking of each other—the awed recognition that we are, each one of us, a universe.

I am sure that every one of us has a similar shower of associations, for there is no way to live to sixty, or even twenty-eight, without some meaningful and meaning-challenging exposure to our medical system, to generous and competent and harried and mediocre physicians, nurses wise and blasé, plodding and inspired counselors and therapists. But why bother to make a combined anthology, especially when these stories fly right past one another in real life? Maybe because there are so very many stories. For this painful mismatch of expectations and needs drives us all to speech—and there is a lot of that speech. Listen in as patients compare notes on the internet or in support groups. The social implications of that mismatch are an amplification of personal anguish, a precipitous rise in litigation and a paralyzing level of chronic mistrust.

The difficult question is how much if any of this chronic friction can be changed? How much is structural, the result of our crazy quilt healthcare system? Social—the result of professional training and incommensurate social expectations? Psychological? Whatever the cause, how much is intransigent? Intractable?

Why is it so difficult for patients to listen to their doctors' stories, to accept the walk-on parts they are given in the doctor's heroic battle against

DISEASE? Why is it so hard for physicians to spend even five minutes in the absolutely unique reality of any given patient's experience of sickness?

Thomas Graboys in his book *Life in the Balance,* which describes his own experience of Parkinson's disease and Lewy body dementia, quotes Anatole Broyard's desire that his doctor "would *brood* on my situation for perhaps five minutes, that he would give me his whole mind just once . . . ." Graboys, himself a physician, and one noted for his own holistic approach and attention to patients, recognizes the enormous burden this expectation places on physicians: "How do you give yourself over to hundreds and still function as a physician, a spouse, and a parent?" But as a patient, he also says, "That is why, as Broyard says, we cannot expect our physicians to suffer with us. But we can expect them to move out from behind the technology and pharmacology to connect with us briefly, to genuinely share, for a moment, our pain and anguish."

In her memoir, Amy Silverstein describes how she decided never to confuse long-term camaraderie between her and her physicians with friendship. She didn't want to be on a first name basis with the person who might in time tell her that she was dying and that there was nothing he could do to stop it. Underneath that resistance, there is of course a pervasive need— and a genuine and humane reality—in these decades-long relationships that is life-giving. Part of the process she goes through in this memoir is to claim it, to release herself from the ways she diminishes her own world.

For when we talk about doctor-patient or nurse-patient realities, we often don't discuss as well the powerful centripetal pull of illness, how it can absorb not only the self of the person experiencing it but also the selves of those around her. If we read patients' memoirs, doctors and nurses appear, often at life-defining times. Opening one door, shutting another, they march through unscathed. The drama is essentially solitary and metaphysical. It is about what happens when we find ourselves alone in a dramatically transformed world where nothing means what it once did, where simple words like 'body,' 'tomorrow,' 'normal' are filled with spaces we tumble through again and again without warning.

And yet that word *pathography* shocks me in this context. Who is defining here? And why? For I do hear in most memoirs of illness a profound blessing story, a rising to the enormity and magnanimity of mortality. But it is an intense journey to enter even for the time it takes to read a book (just trying reading a few back to back). Who among us could do it twenty times a day, even for five minutes at a time? Especially if we were trained to see it as the abnormal, the pathological, the contradiction of our own *raison d'être*.

Why *is* it so important that we can hear the stories of people with different roles, different social locations as taking place in the same reality?

This is actually a very tricky question in medicine and healthcare. Professionalization is usually defined by having a specialized body of knowledge, a systemic way of looking at the world that is different from 'common' knowledge, 'common' sense. This different way of looking at the world, however, derives its value from the *social* function that profession plays—and that social function must, by definition, have a common denominator. Within a profession, the intrinsic value of the knowledge system itself is usually used as the proof of the profession's social standing. However, in the world at large, it is the importance of the general human condition it addresses (illness, death) and its success at meeting its *social* function (to relieve us in some way of this fear and suffering) that provides the status of the profession. Medicine and healthcare are important because they help us as a society live longer and less painfully with illness. They are measured by how successfully they address our social fear of our inescapable mortality and vulnerability to disease. No other profession comes so close to what it means to be human, to be ourselves. The stories we hear here, the stories we find in ourselves, tell us something, often more than we might like to know, about the essential meaning of life. No wonder a careless word by a busy and abstracted physician can turn a world topsy-turvy. The worst part of it often is that the other person didn't even notice.

Professions define themselves to some extent by talking about people in different terms, a different language, within their system of knowledge and action than they do outside it. We have the patient (bearer of suffering) and the doctor (wielder of knowledge) not Herb and Jessie. And the way Jessie describes Herb when in his hearing and when alone with her colleagues may not only be quite different but irreconcilable with the way Herb understands himself. The stories he tells, at home, away from the smells of the clinic or hospital, may be equally incomprehensible to *Dr.* Jessie. This distance, this disjuncture, is a good measure of the level of social distrust and chronic discord. In some areas of our life, this disjuncture is not crucial, but it is in healthcare because we are, finally, dealing with care, with our society's response to core human vulnerability, core social contracts. It is, always, ultimately, about *us*.

In this anthology, we are suggesting by our use of categories that cut across professional divides, that associate patients' realities and doctors' realities around common themes, that the more the way we talk *to* each other and the way we talk *about* each other are congruent, the more we begin to heal our system, hold our whole. This suggestion goes for everyone. If we want our doctor or nurse to share our reality, even for five minutes, we must be willing to share theirs too. The categories that we use in this anthology—immediate experience, boundaries, long-term relationships, defining experience: the power of words, errors, growing in our roles, and changing places—apply to all of us.

The authors who have sent their work to us are also interested in addressing this divide, or they wouldn't have submitted. On both sides, they had important experiences they wanted to share. In "The Gift," Matthew Smith writes forthrightly about what it felt like as a physician to accept valid criticism from a patient, while David Page in "Burr Holes in the Heart" writes as a surgeon and a brother about the devastating impact of negative outcomes on all involved. In "My Doctor and I," Nancy Brandwein explores the complexity of a relationship that has lasted as long as her marriage. Nina Gaby writes personally about her own experience of commitment and burn-out in "The Inventories We Keep" and serves as scribe for a group of residents at Second Spring, a transitional facility for people transitioning from the state psychiatric hospital to the community, who were inspired by the web publication of her essay to write their own. Gerri Luce's powerful memoir "The Fine Line Between Love and Insanity" describes inhabiting both sides of the experience of mental illness, as patient and as therapist, and the role of writing in helping her bridge these two roles, claim this one reality.

We do note that almost all the work submitted, poetry or prose, was memoir. That makes sense since people have very personal bones to pick, thanks to give, and unique existential sense to make. However, one very practical suggestion we make here is that we all use some of the crucial assumptions of fiction rather than memoir, in real life and in reading—and take on the role of the omniscient narrator, graced listener, the one who can bear to enter into other realms of experience, can bear to hold all those points of view in a single story that is more than the story of any one of the people in it.

Who has the time? the tired suffering patient might ask. Or the harried nurse. Or the over-scheduled doctor. Who *doesn't?* If we cannot entertain, even for five minutes, the reality of another, can we ever, truly, do them justice? It takes very little time—but it does require a liberating moment of full, free attention. It does release us into a healing, humane and ultimately mysterious *more*. Try it as you read here. Try it the next time you are in an examining room.

This anthology is the result of two disparate calls for submissions. One was directed to nurses, physicians, therapists and other healthcare professionals: *The Patient Who Changed My Life*, and was first published as a web anthology. A subsequent call was directed toward patients and their responses and was originally titled, "The Doctor or Nurse Who for Better (or Worse) I Can't Forget." It is important that we didn't ask for expository essays, for people's responses to the health system as a whole, to doctors or nurses (or patients) as categories, but for a personal experience that had a direct, lasting impact on one's own life. We were interested in reflection on that experience.

As could be expected, we received substantially more submissions for the second call. It took awhile to decide on a title for the combined collection, but when *View from the Bed ❈ View from the Bedside* came to us, it felt right since it did seem that these disparate points of view had a common meeting point—the sick bed (or examining table or imaging machine). I had a strong desire, and still do, to call it *Under One Roof* because our focus is on what holds these disparate, often achingly, frighteningly, sometimes humorously— and always stubbornly—different points of view together is the irreducible reality of illness and death. Sooner or later, every one of us will find ourselves on a sick bed and, if we love, at its side as well. Death, illness, essential vulnerability *and its care* is there, always the real heart of healthcare, whether its pulse is steady, erratic, slow.

Pauline Chen writes fascinatingly in her memoir *Final Exam* about how doctors' attitudes toward mortality are shaped by their temperaments, their training and their practice—and how these attitudes both help in the provision of care and also increasingly isolate physicians from their own inner life and from their patients when disease can't be vanquished.

Stories of medical success fit, quite comfortably, with a little carping here, a little quipping and clipping there, under one roof. It is the other stories, the ones we really need to hear and to tell that interest us here. The ones either the doctor or nurse doesn't have time to hear or the patient doesn't have the heart or stomach for, the ones that let us know what we look like to each other when we don't feel we're on the same team or even in the same game. And not only the BIG ones, but also the little, damaging interchanges that take place a hundred times a day.

If we're interested in what people find difficult to say, or to hear, in each other's presence—where does that leaves us as publishers committed to finding the We in Them, the Us in You? This was my first uncomfortable insight when, after having collected and ordered these interesting selections, I tried to imagine what groups of people could read this book together and join in conversation through it. Doctors, and often nurses, really don't want to spend extended time in their patients' often narcissistic worlds. The same is true for patients. They don't want to wander through their doctors' minds in which they play, at best, a walk-on part. The point seems obvious—and as understandable as the daughter or son of any age putting their hands over their ears when a parent decides to share his or her sexual quandaries, peccadilloes, however ancient. *Too much information!* So much desire to be heard.

For we also note that the people who wrote here all hungered, for a variety of reasons, to be in conversation with a world that had not fully understood them. And it is people like that we wish to reach with this anthology, who can then quietly, one by one, share it with someone else whose story could fit in here, who would welcome a common roof.

We want to reach the physician or nurse who can feel that an important opportunity to create a more caring and trusting connection, to participate in a healing story, was lost and they don't know exactly what went wrong but they know it matters. We want to reach physicians who are tired of dreading their time with their patients because they always feel they are walking on eggshells, that their words are misunderstood, that the expectations of them are unrealistic or completely off-base and so are the interpretations. And the ones who get it, whose relations with their patients are good, but are tired of seeing these failed opportunities all around them.

We want to reach the nurse and therapist who know they have something important to add to this conversation about care—and some of it involves speaking truth to a resistant structure, and some of it involves opening their hearts, and some of it involves holding people accountable too.

And we want to reach the patients who may be getting tired of feeling let down or dismissed—who know that the stories they find themselves telling about their doctors or nurses are too stylized, too predictable and that some part of them wants a completely different tone, a different dialogue, doesn't know how to get it started, but does know it is never too soon to start. And that it begins right here.

For this anthology we did not go out and seek the very best, the last word, in previously published medical writing. We have some beautiful writing here by some very accomplished writers; most of it hasn't been published before. Indeed, with many of the pieces, I'm not sure they were written originally with publication in mind, rather from a strong drive to understand, to absorb, to in some way right a vision of the world. We put out two calls, one to professionals and another to that group that excludes none of us, those who know the sickbed. We looked at what we received over the transom, selecting good, solid, heartfelt writing from writers who are not that different from you or me, who face similar events, are driven to speech by similar frustrations and joys. This is a roof that has room for you too. This is a conversation that has room for your voice, your insights, your truth. *And more.*

For when we reach people through this anthology, we want to get them, whether from the bed or from the bedside, to start imagining a story that can hold, generously, the subjective realities of everyone in the room—the patient, the nurse, the doctor, the grieving mother, the bewildered daughter—can see them as part of a complex whole, can feel all these multiple interpretations adding up compassionately, at times comically, at times profoundly, to something larger and richer than any one of their separate stories and feel they themselves are an essential part of that more.

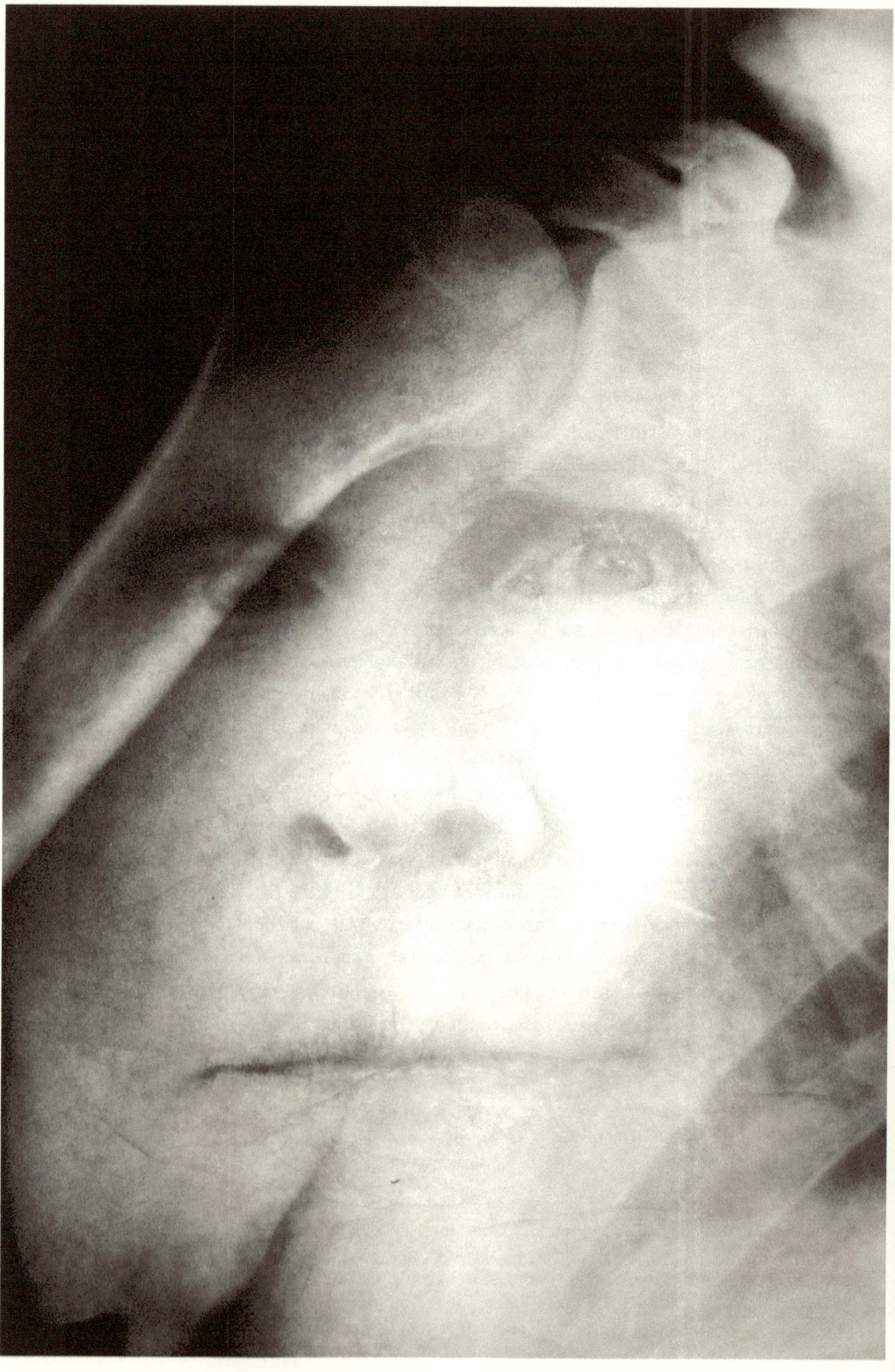

I
IMMEDIATE EXPERIENCE

PAUL HOSTOVSKY

PSALM

I give myself to you, my
anesthesiologist—
for you I have fasted,
for you disrobed,
donned the humble
johnny that closes in the back,
climbed up into the narrow
bed on wheels,
hugging my novel,
waiting for you to come
with your clipboard and questions
I've already answered
three times already,
because you are infinitely
thorough because we are
talking about my future pain here.
The thing about future pain is
you can always count on it being there.
Thank god for you, my
anesthesiologist,
and your technology
for predicting the body's weather
and sheltering me from it
with your little concoction,
this wonderful confection
you're whipping up for me now
and pouring into my IV
as you recite the names for me
of its secret ingredients:

Hydrocodone,
Acetaminophen,
and a dash of something extra special
whose name is nearly
as unpronounceable
and beautiful as your own,
O Everyanesthesiologist.
And now I feel you gently
relieving me of my fiction
and reading glasses
and the caterpillars
of your eyebrows are
already beginning their sweet
metamorphosis.

THE NURSE'S OFFICE

I like it here. I don't feel sick
but I don't feel good exactly either.
I like it when you ask me questions
about how I feel and since when.
I don't know how to answer them
exactly. It hurts here, and here. It feels
good to be touched and puzzled over.
I think if anyone can solve the puzzle
you can. I like your stethoscope
on my skin. And your eyebrows
coming together over my underlying
condition. I like your new thermometer
in my ear, but I liked the old one better
under my tongue, with its promise
of you returning in 3 minutes to read it.
Now I sit here in this chair with my
symptoms while you write at your desk
all the way over there. Out in the hall
it's quiet. The only sound's the sweep
of the long broom—Tony our custodian
pushing his way up the infinitely tessellating
checkered floor with his jutting elbows and rose
tattoo climbing. The coast is clear. See you
tomorrow, I say, and slip back out
into infinity before you look up.

MARIETTE LANDRY

FREEDOM TRAIL

In an oversized surgical gown and gloves
not made for my mother's hands, she stood

out among the other interns, watching
the first amputations. These,

she once told me, were hardest, even
though she'd grown used to the sound of the saw

through a femur, the sudden jump of blood
from a forgotten artery left unclamped.

Last night a friend called from New York. She wants
me to keep an eye out for her husband, who is somewhere

in Boston with a woman she tries to picture: light-haired,
she imagines, smiling, her opposite in every way.

Go to the museums, she tells me; the woman will treat him
as a tourist. The Aquarium, Old Ironsides, the North End.

If it's sunny, the Freedom Trail. She wants to know
how they look together, if his hand fits easily

into hers. And I think of my mother, who even now,
after years of practice, still finds herself unnerved

by certain things: the women my brother brings home
for dinner, jokes told to jar her in the doctors' lounge,

the sight of a single leg, detached,
whole, moving slowly past her, cradled

oddly in the arms of a stranger.

ZOË LOSADA

SHADOWS

In my life
spent in the shadow of your death
I have discovered the healing rites:
the shape of hope in
reflected sunlight,
the laying on of hands,
baths in the water
of steeping purple flowers,
the long river of prayer.

But like the most bitter betrayal,
I know that
one day
at last
the harsh rumble of your
wounded heart will stop.
And I cannot bear it.

It is the process that matters.
The slow steps up the mountain
that overlooks our days,
the joyful dance of the dreadlocked
orderly to the beat of the machine
that pumped your heart.

He carried us to a life
I had not imagined for you, my son.
I could not bear it
But I did.

And now,
years later
you are alive
in a moment between past and future
peeling oranges and planting flowers,
on a day of sunshine
and shadows.

PAULA SERGI

SUDDEN WRINKLE

The woman in 319, from some small town up north
sits alone and sobs for the first time
now that her husband has turned around to go back home
to the kids after driving all day, back roads to
highway to interstate, through the maze of one-ways
and round-abouts, past the capital, to the University.

She's been put in the ancient unit called "infirmary,"
in a dark room with a crack in the floor,
a bathroom down the hall, a view of the other wing.
She's got a bad prognosis and now she's got me,
a brand new nurse with a new uniform, maybe turquoise,
maybe pink, but surely polyester, and almost to my knees.

Twenty-two and what I bring to the job
is an independent study in pharmacology:
when to mix beer with tequila and pot,
how to pad my stomach lining with bread
or mac and cheese before a night out.
My penmanship is crisp, dotted I's, crossed T's,

pretty good grammar when I ask her for samples
in a cup. I bring a willingness to please, to say always
the right thing. But what can I say to her worries
about treatment, a metal cage with radium
implanted between her legs? She wonders will it hurt,
will she feel the need to urinate all day?

Will she see her kids this weekend, or see them grow
past summer? I have no answers. What I do is bring her water
in a plastic pitcher, some bleach-scented towels, straighten
a sudden wrinkle in her sheets. What I do is sit there,
listening to her rehearse her lines, rearrange her view point
from the living to the almost dead.

PATRICIA KETT

END OF LIFE

Her mouth stretches wide
pulling her shriveled skin
taut across her boney face,
eyes clenched shut
neck hyperextended,
the face of a scream
without sound
energy emitting
from bone, muscle and nerve.

I see it when I enter her room.
I feel it when I suction the mucus
from the tube blocking her sound,
when I turn her to clean
the dried excrement from her back,
rub the cream into her wasted flesh
position her with pillows
cover her.

Only then,
her mouth closes,
muscles relax
her body is silent
until the next time, or
until her final rest
which we have
so successfully
postponed.

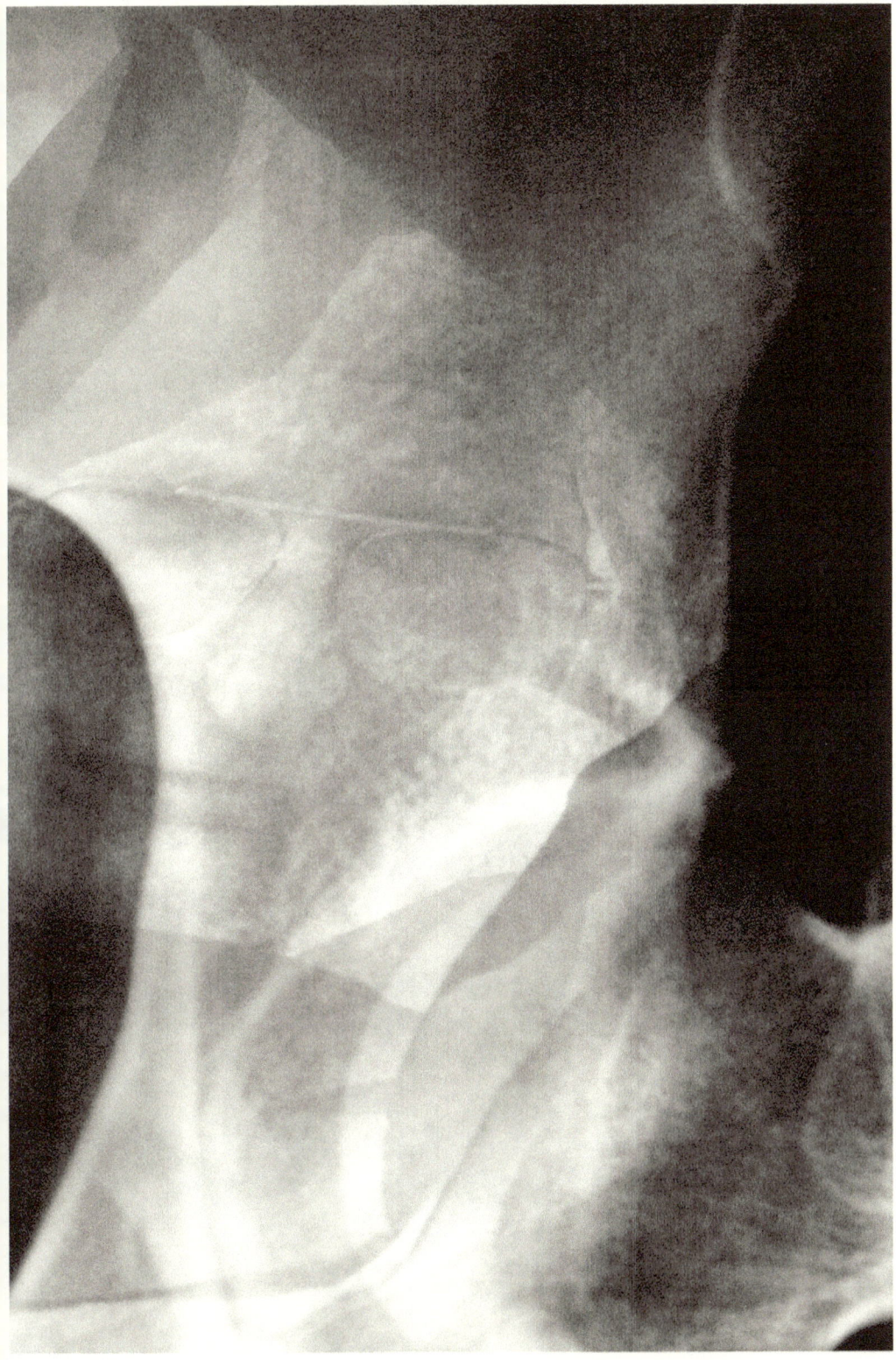

KATHLEEN M. KELLEY

IF I COULD PAINT THEM
For Susan and Karl

The curtain has been drawn
around the bed, the light so dim,
when I enter the hospital room,
I think for a moment
I might be too late.

But I look behind the curtain
and see the man asleep in the recliner,
wearing blue hospital pajamas
and facing the wall.
The woman is in the bed,
her head at its foot
so that she too, sleeping
in her street clothes, faces the wall.
And just for a minute
I become confused
about which one is the patient:
they have pushed the bed and the recliner
as close together as possible
and sleep now, looking somehow pleased
with themselves,
and holding hands.

Indeed, they are up against a wall,
And yet, if I could paint them,
I would not paint them as prisoners of any cruel fate
that could rob them only of time,
for which they care little.
I would paint them as children
happy just being together.
in spite of all that has happened,
in spite of all that is to come.

CLAY

When Monica places the baby ceremonially in my arms, Amy locks her knees like gates and quickly positions herself so she can stand up in my lap and face out. She wears a red jumper, a white blouse, long striped athletic socks in bright shades of blue and purple, and a tiny pair of sneakers the color of goldenrod. She is four months old. Her two moms and I sit down on hard dark chairs and a couch in the conference room in the hospital's radiation oncology department. It is five months since the September 11 terrorist attacks, the day before Valentine's Day. I love holding her, love her vanilla bean smell and the bald spot on the back of her head, but feel a little distracted from the careful listening I want to do.

Grace, Amy's other mom, is my patient. Today she wears an oversized t-shirt with an American flag on the front in the shape of a huge heart. She tells me what I already know, that she is no longer in remission. Not only is the cancer still in her lungs, it is also in her liver and her brain. She has resumed chemotherapy, a protocol less toxic than the one she endured when Monica was pregnant. Grace insists that Dr. Mannan be completely honest with her, so she knows there is only a ten percent chance she will be alive a year from now.

When I comment on the sadness that must permeate their lives, Grace's reply surprises me. "To tell you the truth," she says, "I have never been so happy, so much at peace." Indeed, her face shines. Her disability application has been approved, she is building a high chair in her basement for Amy, and her mother's upcoming visit will end a long period of estrangement between them. Not only that, but they have just mailed paper work that will make Amy Grace's legally adopted child. The baby bounces on my lap with her knees still locked.

Grace is recording her reflections in three keepsake notebooks: one for her mother, one for Monica, and one for Amy. The one for Amy is composed of letters she wants Amy to read when the time is right: *Starting School, Getting Your Period, Falling in Love, Figuring Out About Alcohol,*

Leaving Home. In braver moments, she is working on a piece called *The Mom You Don't Remember,* as well as her personal reflections on dying.

Monica reaches into the diaper bag and brings out a round, dark green wooden box. It is painted in tiny pink flowers curled tightly at the tips of their long, graceful stems. We go ahead with our plan to cut a ceremonial lock of Grace's hair (before any more falls out) to put in the box, another keepsake for Amy. I have come prepared with scissors. When I snip the lock from the back of Grace's neck, the scissors make a bright, crisp sound. We smile. Believe it or not, we are having a good time.

I am also prepared with a package of clay. "Is it time for this now?" I ask, and they nod. Leaving them to wait for me, I walk to the staff lunch room. There, I cut the clay in two with a plastic knife. Then I heat each half on a paper towel in the microwave for a minute, until it rises like a biscuit. Slowly, I flatten each one with my hand, patting it from the center out, as if I were rolling out a pie crust, until I have two warm, smooth spongy pancakes.

When I return, Grace presses each of her hands, one at a time, into the warm clay, while Monica and I look on, smiling and pressing our own hands against hers so the impressions will be as clear as possible. Then Monica holds the wriggling baby over the clay. I press each of her tiny hands into the clay inside Grace's prints so that the big hand will be holding the little one. She shrieks and balks as we hold her still, uncurl her fingers, and press hard. The impressions are perfect. In twenty-four hours the clay will be dry.

During the next year, I meet with Grace often enough to feel quite close to her. Eventually, she becomes too sick to come into the hospital any more. Her care is transferred to hospice. I miss our meetings, understand how fragile she is, and decide to make a home visit. A woman with a full face and thin lips lets me in. She is Eva, an old friend who is taking care of Grace in the last weeks of her life, and she leads the way upstairs to a room where Grace lies in a hospital bed. Then she discreetly disappears. It is hot and humid in the house. Grace has no shirt on. Her pendulous breasts rest on her stomach, as if they have just been emptied. I can tell she is glad to see me again. She makes a little joke about being shirtless, says she hopes it doesn't matter since we're all women. Grace is usually very direct, so her comment does not surprise me. Still, it takes me a moment to adjust to seeing her this way. I have never made a home visit to a dying patient, and I have no idea what sort of professional boundary is appropriate.

Grace seems both herself and not herself. Much of her body has wasted away; she does her best to focus through a fog of morphine. Still, when our eyes meet the gaze holds, and when she speaks, her voice is the same—honest, funny, wise.

What do you say to someone who is dying? I feel awkward, aware how little experience I have with this, except for my mother's death. I ask how she is feeling and watch her face for a sign she hears me, hoping the question does not strike her under the circumstances as ridiculous. After a moment her face breaks out in a broad smile, and she says she is actually doing pretty well. There is a pause, then she says that every single face she looks into—and I especially recall her use of the word "single"—seems full of love, and she can't imagine anything better than that. I see in my mind the faces of the people she loves, at least the ones I know—the baby, of course, and Monica, who must be at once both overwhelmed and distracted by the need to make a living and take care of Alice.

Eva has come upstairs now to see if Grace needs anything. Grace says her mouth is dry. Eva reaches for a tube of gel and offers it to me with a question on her face. I understand she is offering to let me put some gel on my finger and smooth it around Grace's mouth. It is the kind of act Eva must perform a dozen times a day. I am unprepared for the gesture, confused again about the professional boundaries that usually apply in my work but don't seem to apply here. So I shrug my shoulders and shake my head as if to say I don't quite understand how all this works, which is true. Rescuing me, Eva moistens Grace's mouth with the gel, then leaves us alone again.

I am glad for the silence that envelops us as Grace drifts in and out of consciousness. Once in awhile she says something that lets me know she is aware I'm still there. Once she reassures me that she is still "there" no matter how it looks. I am struck by how gracious she is to give me this feedback even as she lies dying. There is a lump in my throat and a bee in my belly. I have no idea how to be helpful. I only know I needed to see her this one last time to say good-bye.

After a while, as if from a great distance, Grace says she is hungry. She says this as if hunger surprises her, tickles her in some way. I tell her I will let Eva know, then go downstairs to ask if Eva if she can bring up something to eat.

When Eva returns I am surprised to see that she has brought an orange, which she hands to me. Grace has shared a lot of her writing with me, and once she wrote about oranges—how they were God's gift and how she loved their taste almost as much as she had once loved alcohol, how she would hoard them as a child and eat them by the bagful. Holding the orange in my hand, I remind Grace of the piece she wrote, which makes her smile. She reminds me that she expects me to read it at her funeral, which makes me smile. Then I surprise myself by asking her if she knows how to peel an orange with a spoon. There is a twinkle in her eye as she shakes her head no. I ask Eva if she can bring up a spoon, which she quickly does, then raises the bed up so Grace is in a semi-sitting position.

I hold the orange up so Grace can see it clearly. I pierce the skin with the tip of the spoon and watch as oil poofs into the air as if from an atomizer, suffusing the air in the tight room with a sharp fragrance. Carefully, I probe with the spoon the space between the peel and the fruit, moving slowly in a circular fashion with an almost ratcheting motion, the way you do when peeling an apple so the skin comes off in a one long dancing spiral. Grace lets out a giggle, and a sigh of pleasure. The orange is very ripe, even a little overripe, so I am making a mess. There is juice running down my arm as I pull open the fruit and raise a piece to Grace's open mouth. Eva helps her to lean forward. With an openhearted smile, she takes a fragment of the fruit into her mouth where she savors it for a moment, then utters the one word *delicious*.

This effort exhausts her, and when she lies back down she seems to sink more deeply into the bed and to retreat into a sleep that carries her away to a place I cannot go. When I kiss her good-bye, she barely responds.

At her funeral service the next week I bring a large basket of oranges to share. Alice plays with them on the floor to everyone's delight, rolling them like balls.

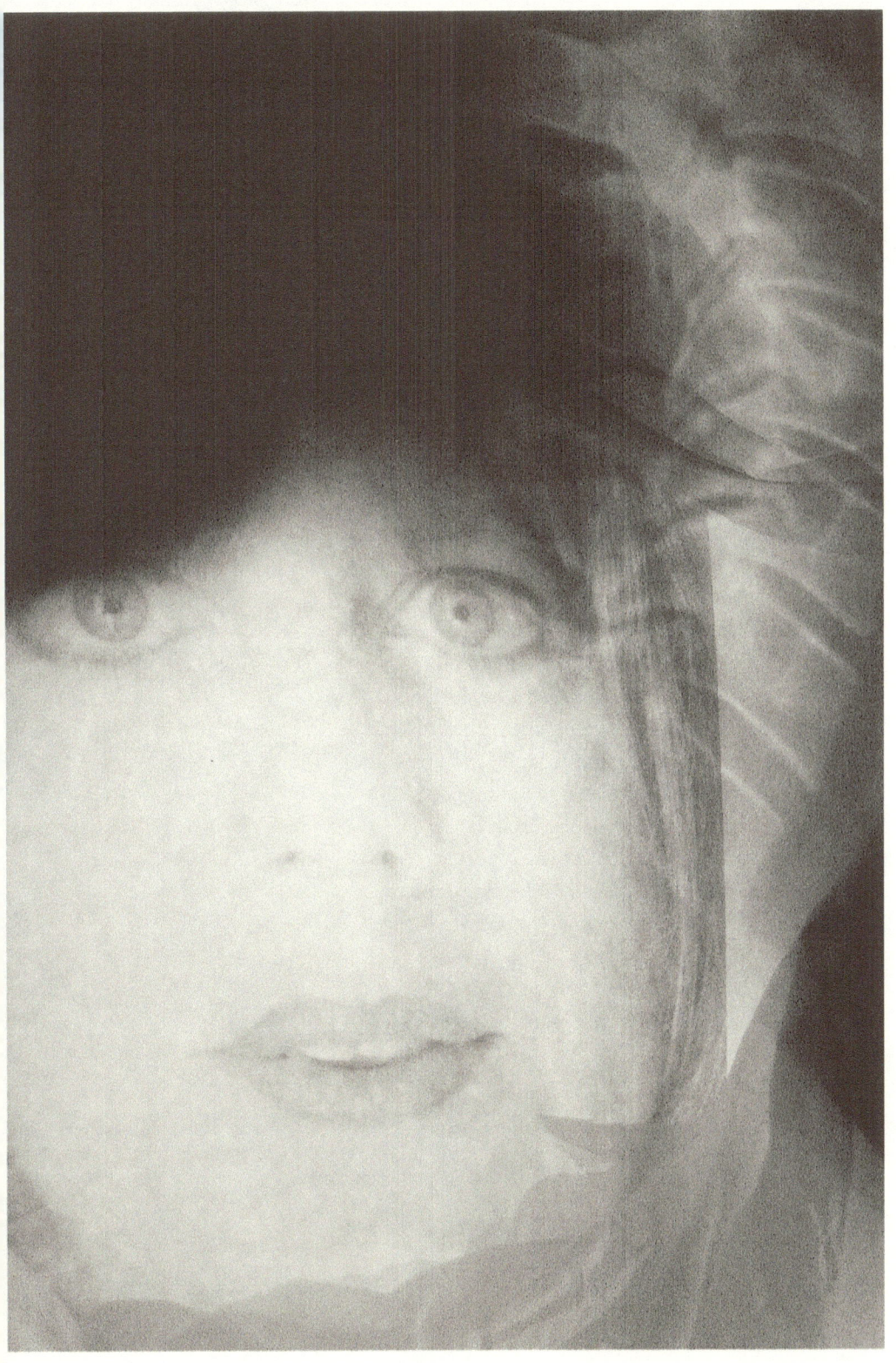

MOLLY O'DELL

BETTY WAS A CONCERT PIANIST

I'm called to the farm. Betty quit eating.
Her son and his wife feel helpless.
When I lead myself to Betty's room, I pass
her Steinway covered with dust. She's curled
on her side in the dark, musty curtains closed
to late day sun. She admits she won't eat,
then chokes out the secret. When I confirm
her impaction and explain what I must do,
she submits to my instructions. While I dig
out the contents of her large intestine, I learn
she teaches with Chopin's etudes and likes
playing Liszt and Brahms from the portfolio
on the piano. When I've finished, she whispers
"Thank you" into the pillow and I close the door
on her dignity. The couple make supper
in the kitchen in their socks, barn boots
left outside the door. After my report
I look at photos of Betty and her husband
and of Betty in a concert gown. Before I leave,

I thank them for the glass of sherry.

EATING PLACENTA: A FOUND POEM
From research in response to a patient's request to eat her placenta

Most mammals eat what's
formed in union egg and sperm
baby's sibling friend dead twin

interface of mom and fetus
lungs and kidneys bridge to life

Hungarian women bite placenta
Chinese dry eat natal jing

some now freeze for late consumption
those that rip it out are thieves

placentophagia raises eyebrows
chew it raw fry with onions—

roast it whole or make lasagna
bake and dry encapsulate

allay depression sooth the pain
shrink the womb enhance lactation

hold the cord once its been cut
print the image on a page

blot resembles full grown tree.

FIRST HOUSE CALL

"Come quick and see about the boy,"
he says. My ad boasts of house calls,
so I follow the man I recognize
as the Ferris wheel operator
at the summer carnival
over the river and up the mountain,
about half way to a hollow
off the road. There's an entrance
to what, exactly, I cannot tell.
I go in through a framed
entry to a cave
that stands for a house
and is clearly the home
for the mom and dad, and the boy.
Waiting in his jury-rigged chair, a pair
of blue eyes search mine, and he lifts
a crooked hand to shake. His buckled
spine allows his head to rest
on his hips. A twisted face
blows air as loud as a wind
tunnel. His tangled body defies
exam. Saw a doctor thirty years
ago. Science offered nothing,
so they've been making do.
Now the work of breathing's
too painful to watch,
so I arrive with nothing
much to offer but a few drugs
to ease him and them and me.

SKY WALKER

He needs a prescription to help him sleep
and needs that dose of coke and booze
to let him do his job—twenty stories up
on rusted beams in another city.
He feels crazy coming down
from hours on a ledge of near falls.
His shift crew thinks the downers take off
the edge they need to balance. He knows this stuff
spikes his pressure, reminds me I treated
his wife's busted eardrum last week. But he needs
the work, needs the guts to go to work—
one month on, then two months off to plough
the ground, patch Daddy's fence, and track
the T-ball game his boy is pitching.
He needs a fix of normal for the day.

SOMATIC COMPLAINT

Worn as an empty coin sack,
she returns to the office
for itching. The salve I prescribed
hasn't helped. I can only guess
the sounds that start her days,
if she sets the table before eating,
the titles of the books in her trailer,
or what she feels on a moonless night.

My office note mentions the death
of her mother, the same visit the itching
started.

The skin at the base of her neck
is a washboard.

She asks *if it came from*
Mama gripping me around
the neck when I lifted her into the bath
every day.

MAXINE SUSMAN

CATSKILL REGIONAL ER, 3:30 A.M.

Behind a curtain a man gives his history.
Shot in the stomach, '87, scarring, internal damage.
Then the RN keeps talking, upbeat, one guy to another,
Hate to do this to you buddy keep swallowing that stuff I need a straight shot
don't want to hit the lungs you're not gonna like this but bear with me fella—
in seconds threads a tube down the man's throat.

Through the night towards dawn, gurgling, wet coughs, retching
but no cry, no moan. A belch; a hoarse *Excuse me.*
At the foot of his bed on folding chairs meant for significant others
two enormous prison guards drink coffee, from time to time
offer brief encouragement. *Hang in there. Stay the course.*
One toys with his bunch of keys, the other says
he hopes they'll stay a few more hours,
he's in no rush, they'll make overtime.

GARY YOUNG

THE TUMOR IS SMALL

This tumor is smaller than the last one, he said. I'm going to cut it out, and then do my best to stitch you back together. He leaned forward, and pulled a blade across my leg. Smoke rose from the open wound as he cauterized the tiny veins, and while he worked, he spoke to me. Every body is a machine, he said. When they break, I fix them. But there's an art to it, he said. We have to coax some kind of magic or luck out of the body. Some patients die, he said, and others find a way to beat the odds. That's what I expect of you. Do you know what I'm saying, he asked? I nodded while my breath kept pace with the morphine drip. Good, he said, and he put his knee on the table for a better purchase. I watched my leg jump and fall as he jerked on the sutures. That should hold, he said, but you're going to feel it for a while.

SYLVIE TERESPOLSKI

MY SISTER'S DREAMS AND DR. ADAM APPLE, THE SHRINK

"It's either that you can't stand being married, or can't stand being married to him." I finally commanded the courage to tell my sister June she needed to see a shrink. I was tired of being the only repository of her constant *qveching*, and shifts into bouts of depression about her eighteen-year long-suffering relationship with Edward, her spouse. Often called Edward the Terrible, as my sister fancied herself a historian.

"May," she said, "What do you know? You have your Jewish laws, your *sheitel* that covers your gorgeous curly hair, your so-called absolutes."

I grinned hoping to relax her. "I know a lot," I said. "I know enough to be happy that we weren't born in September or October because Mom would have thought those could be good names. At least we were born in the months of May and June. April would have been okay. You know, I bet that's where you get your restlessness—from Mom."

"So, you admit, I've got restlessness."

"I'm giving something a name. Admitting, I'm not. I'm giving it a name like restlessness because you're my sister. If I had to give the name to someone else, maybe I would call it *craziness, not normal, bewitched*. For you I call it restlessness."

June changed the subject or maybe it wasn't such a change of subject. "I couldn't do what you just did."

"Which was?" As if I didn't know.

"Go to Israel and pray every day for forty days at the Kotel that you would find a husband instead of going to Tiberias or swimming in the Dead Sea, or night-clubbing in Tel-Aviv."

"What couldn't you do? Pray? Go to the same place every day?"

"Both," she said this "restless" sister of mine so close and so far from me. Moderation was not in her mindset—in her framework. When a subject was to be learned, she read five books instead of the requisite two. When a sport was to be mastered, she devoted four hours a day of practice and often wound up with some piece of her body that needed mending. When there was a friendship or a cause to nurture, the word "limit" became unknown to her. Once when we were on a vacation with the kids at the shore, I caught her at the skateboarding park, well-padded at the knees, and a securely fastened helmet on her head. She outlasted and outworked the nine year old. Her kids seemed to take their mother in stride better than I did and I marveled that they still had egos after doing anything competitive with her. When I was starting to reconnect with my Judaism and going to Torah classes, my niece and nephew begged me not to tell her. I assured them that this bit of news I could tell her—her fight against religion was fierce—as fierce as anything she fought for.

Sometimes when I was deep into my prayers—yes, as a woman, I could be *deep into my prayers* because I was "Modern Orthodox"—my thoughts would wander from my affirmations to Eloheim, to questions about where her nuttiness came from. After all, I was just two years older than June and I heard the same Martin Buber quotes that Mom insisted we have with our tuna melt dinners. Sometimes we got Hamburger Helper and TV dinners but mostly it was tuna melt and Martin Buber:

"Play is the exultation of the possible."

"Solitude is the place of purification."

"The world is not comprehensible, but it is embraceable: through the embracing of one of its beings."

The last one was particularly meaningful to me as a sixteen year old because I decided I was in love with Richard Fogel and it sounded as though Buber was telling me that the next time I got together with Richard an embrace was definitely in order.

Pop would come home from the jewelry store where he specialized in watch repairs, eat the tuna melt, drink a schnapps, and head for the chair in the living room with a copy of *The New York Times*. He usually turned to the sports section first and then the crossword puzzle. Only once did I ever hear him say, "How about a steak and some potatoes?" or "Enough with the Martin Buber." He seemed to have the good sense to know that he was better off staying distant from our lives—that Mom would undoubtedly withhold her gratifying, enormous breasts from him should he tread too close to the

triumvirate that ruled the apartment. From Buber and tuna melts, I thought
I learned moderation. June apparently learned excess.

"I think it's both," she said. "I think I can't stand Edward and I can't
stand being married. It doesn't suit me." She hesitated. "I think."

"June, I know I'm not supposed to ask but what did Dr. Apple say?"
She had chosen this therapist because she liked his name. She thought the words
Adam Apple were inspirational. I regarded the therapist/patient relationship
the way some people regard the confessional in the Catholic Church. Sacred,
Holy. You could be smited or smote because asking a question could destroy
whatever they were trying to create.

"He told me to record my dreams, and we would discuss them."

"And?"

"I told him the dream where I wander into ocean with my clothes
on to save Edward, and the dream where I'm not prepared for class and the
teacher is angry with me and I have a heart attack, and the dream where I go
from room to room in a house yet every room is in a different house, and the
dream where I'm picking up Mom on the Jersey Turnpike and not sure where
the exit is and—"

I interrupted. "How many visits have you had? I thought you only
went once."

June said, "I did only go once."

I couldn't resist. "What did he say?"

June said, "If I tell you, isn't that supposed to destroy some magical
thing that could happen in this whole process?"

"I think so," I said tentatively because I knew lying was against
HaShem's law. I also distinctly remembered Buber's "God wants man to
fulfill his commandments as a human being and with the quality peculiar to
human beings." Wasn't it peculiar to human beings to want to know the most
intimate details about others?

"It's not going to matter," June whispered. "All he said was *Hmmm*
and he'll see me next week." June smiled. "Want to meet after my next
session?" I guess her sisterly instinct told her what I was thinking.

It was good to see the spark back in June. The prospect of a divorce
had been hard on her and the children. I hoped and prayed I could get her
to see that bringing a little God into her life might be positive. She hadn't
had it easy this beautiful raven-haired sister of mine who dealt in excess. Her
friends in school hated her because if they were told to turn in a five-page

paper, she would turn in ten pages—her co-workers in social work didn't like her because she seemed to be able to handle more problems in a week than they could handle in a month. Somebody would send her a postal card from Paris; she'd write back a letter in French. And now, her husband had not just become a thorn in her side, but an ogre, a monster, a dangerous Greek god.

We met at *Sophie's Thai Restaurant* after her next session with Dr. Apple. I had insisted on kosher Thai food. "How do you get kosher Thai?" She threw her purse on the table, and sat down with her head in her hands. I signaled to the waitress to bring the usual plates of Pad Thai noodles.

I was walking on eggshells. "Easy," I said. "No pork and no dairy, and Rabbi Solevetchik's approval."

She twirled the noodles rapidly. "So what would Rabbi Solevetchik say about my situation?"

She still wasn't smiling so instead of answering her, I asked a question.

"So how was your visit to Dr. Apple?"

Her voice was low. I had to lean in to hear her. "Well," June said. "I told him my dreams. I told him I was on a raft alone floating down the Amazon with pink dolphins jumping all around me. One lands on the raft and lies down besides me."

"Interesting," I said. "Does it live? What happens?"

"What happens is that the dream ends when this dolphin lies down."

"What about the other dolphins?" I said trying to be nonchalant, picking up my noodles with my chopsticks and looking for Rabbi Solevechik's imprimatur on the menu.

"Forget the dolphins. There's more." June struggled with wrapping the noodles around her fork. It felt to me that she was fighting to go on.

"In another dream, I'm writing a letter of recommendation for Dermot Mulroney and I'm trying to retrieve it from my computer."

"Who?"

"Dermot Mulroney. He's a movie star I once had a crush on. I thought him highly romantic. Just my type."

I put down my chopsticks. "What did your therapist, Dr. Apple, say about that?" I thought I saw her lip quiver.

"Nothing. I kept telling him my dreams. Walking on a one-way street that suddenly becomes two-way and three young men approach me and I wonder what they are going to do. I enter a movie theatre from the forties."

"What was playing?"

She's irritated. "I don't know. These dreams end." She was quiet and had stopped eating, letting the Pad Thai noodles get cold.

"Don't you like the food?" I asked.

"Kosher Pad Thai just doesn't do it for me."

"Can I ask you what therapist Apple said to you?"

Tears welled and, yes, her mascara started to run just like the cliché. "He was really angry with me—annoyed. He told me that he thought I was telling him so many dreams to overwhelm him, to show that he was a bad therapist. I was stunned. I told him that's what I thought he wanted me to do. By understanding a lot of dreams, he could understand a lot of me."

I debated about taking her hand. She seemed so vulnerable but we were never a touchy-feely family.

"Take my advice," I said. "Stop going to this guy. Put him in your therapists-I'll-never-recommend book. Therapists-I-can't-stand."

"What can I do now?" She drew big breaths to control her sobbing; they sounded like hiccups. Fortunately the restaurant was not crowded.

I took a breath. "Do you want to go talk to Mom?"

Mom had developed early Alzheimer's and her particular characteristics were loss of short-term memory. *I did take a shower. No, you didn't take a shower.* But somehow she had this unbelievable memory of moments long passed that some photo, or thought, or musical note could evoke.

June paused her sobbing to take a breath. "He, that bastard shrink, is all those mean people that hated me—that couldn't accept my . . . my . . . "

" . . . irrational exuberance?" I tried.

She snapped back. She had fully conquered her tears. "It's not irrational. It's me. It's who I am. I didn't need him . . . that Adam's Apple guy to be 'overwhelmed.'" She practically spit out the last word. "So are we going?"

"Now?"

"Why not now? Mom won't know what day it is; we won't be interrupting anything; she might not even recognize us."

I refrained from saying something about tempering her need for instant action once a thought had been expressed but I felt this was not the time. Maybe a trip to Mom would bring her some solace.

We drove to the assisted living facility, Sunny Stony Manor, in silence, parked the car, nodded to the receptionist who insisted we sign in although she had seen us at least fifty times before.

"It's required," she said.

June practically spit out the words, "I understand all about 'required.' Required is my middle name."

I worried about Mom seeing June so angry.

"Sign in, and let's go." I said.

Mom was sitting near the window in a chair perfectly upright with a book in hand. Her Alzheimer's started when she was still physically fit; we were unsure of the toll the disease would take on her. She looked up. I thought there was some acknowledgment in her eyes.

"What are you reading?" I asked.

"None of your business," she retorted.

"Okay, Mom," June said as she sat by the side of the bed and took her hand. "I need help. Edward and I fight all the time because we can't agree on anything—on the kids—on my career and I can't find a fucking shrink to help me."

Mama looked frightened. "What do you want from me?"

"Remember how you used to quote Martin Buber and give us words of wisdom?"

"I never quoted Martin Buber."

June and I looked at each other.

Mother grew agitated, stood up and started to shout waving the book in the air. "We're freaks, that's all. Those two bastards got us nice and early and made us into freaks with freakish standards, that's all. We're the tattooed lady, and we're never going to have a minute's peace, the rest of our lives, until everybody else is tattooed too." She raised her fist, then collapsed in her chair.

"Mom, what are you saying? Do you know who I am? Do you know who we are?"

June touched me on the shoulder. "She's quoting Salinger. We forgot she used to quote Salinger. She remembered it word for word from *Franny and Zooey.*"

Before June could say anything else, Mom started to speak again but at a higher pitch. "We're freaks . . . " but seemed too tired to go on.

June said, "She's saying we are who we are and better accept it and everyone else better accept it, too." My sister smiled her bright bigger than sunshine smile.

"So, do you know what you're going to do about Edward?"

"I don't know yet, but I'm going to kill the therapist. But before that I'm going to tell him you can never have too many dreams."

I turned to say good-bye to Mom and kissed her on her papery cheek.

"Don't forget Martin Buber," I told her.

"Never heard of him," she said and turned to the window letting the book she had on her lap slide to the floor.

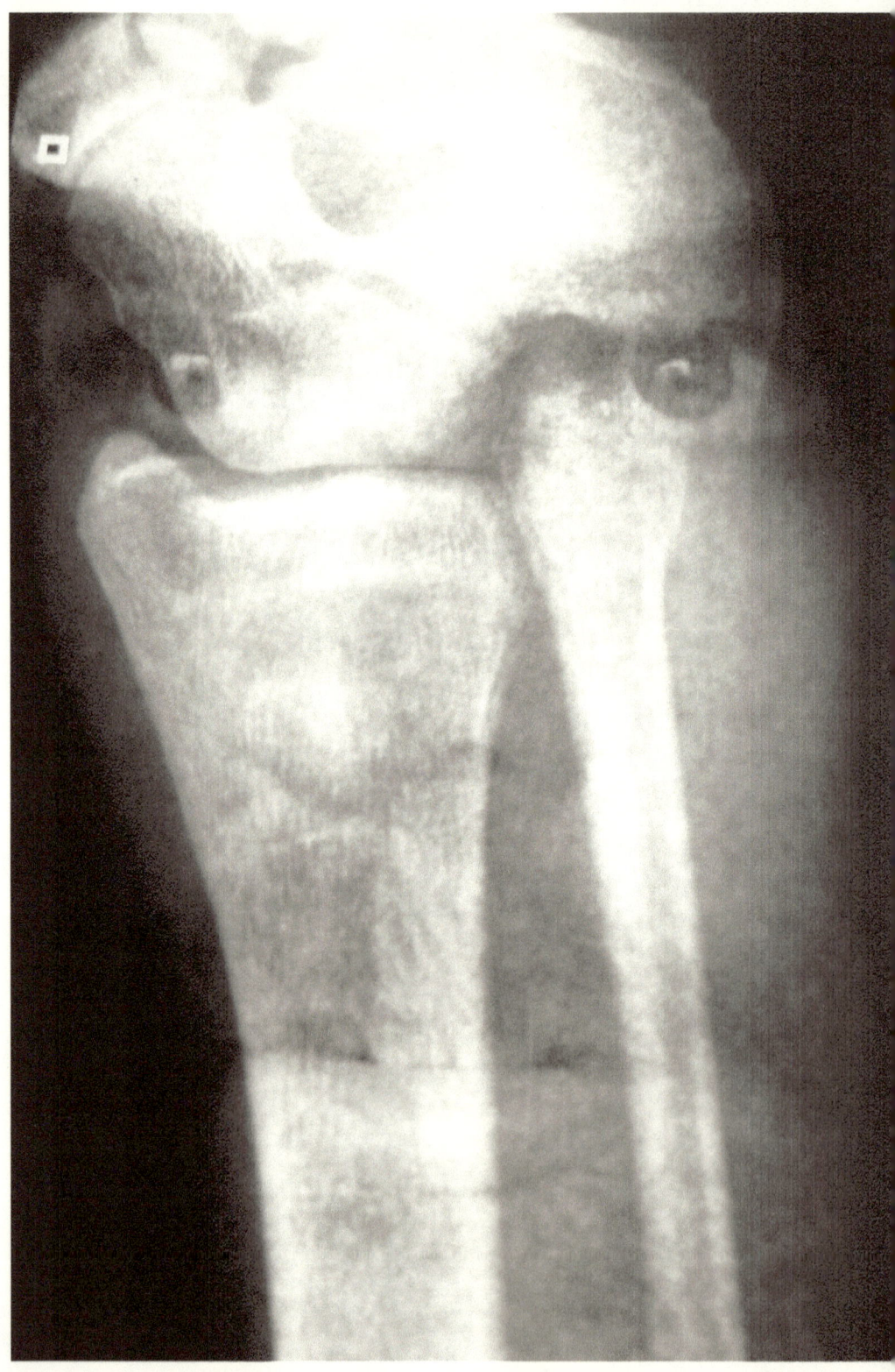

II
BOUNDARIES

KATHLEEN M. KELLEY

WE GO A LITTLE OVER THE HOUR

What pained me most
about my mother's wintry gift
for silent, long suffering,
its loneliness.

My client has written a poem for today
about her own mother, what she remembers:
the warm conversation on their last morning,
the casual way she got in the car,
the truck driver's failed brakes,
his phone call to her family,
(his name, when I ask, gone up in smoke),
the fatal rumor spreading through the schoolyard,
her classmates holding their breath,
the hole burned into the highway,
and afterwards, under her tires,
the daily bump left from a clumsy repair.
What remained, gift of the coroner:
ash burned into a wedding ring.
For her father's sake she scoured it,
though it would not come clean.
And under the bed, Christmas presents,
children's names on unwrapped boxes:
Virginia, Catherine, Peter,
Matthew, Jonathan, Marie.

As we speak it is quiet and her face is flushed.
She is rocking and the clock is ticking.
Memories wrap us like ribbon
and my heart quivers.

People ask how I bear
listening to endless sorrow.
All I can say: it makes a difference.
I can listen to all of it,
and also take the time we need
to read her poem out loud,
though we go a little over the hour.

JOAN PHILLIPS

BOUNDARIES

A tiny magenta blur
Darts across
My waiting room
To wrap arms around my waist
And give me two small pieces of candy
That appear to have been in her warm hand
A long time

The textbooks say
Never touch a client
Never accept a gift
They call this boundaries
Don't do this
Don't do that
Do no harm
Do your best

But boundaries also mean
Containing more than you own heart can keep
Within its small permeable boundary
So I take the candy
Give her a hug back
And our session begins

LESSONS

I actually truly believe
clients come to me
bearing gifts of growth
that I am needing at that moment
and if I figure out what I need
to learn from them, in the process
they will also get what they need.
Not quite this simple, but actually
works most of the time.

So, she comes with this complaint—
although she would not complain
this is her lot in life.
She accepts it, that a man will not
be loving her the way she deserves
to be loved. Has tolerated it even
though she is beautiful and pure
inside and out. Has let this man
be a dust cloud around her radiance.
Feels unable to ask for or get
what she wants in her heart.

I know in my gut what she
needs and deserves. She already
feels better knowing that I know,
though I do not speak it.
Why can't I accept that
within myself as well?
I guess it is time to learn.
Why do I dread this lesson?

RACHEL SQUIRES BLOOM

ISCHEMIC BOWEL, DEMENTIA

Ischemic bowel, dementia,
is typed blackly on the form.
Nowhere do I find a name
to alphabetize. Ah, A Anderson,
F female, born in 1923, here's
the number, code to coax insurance
to pay for surgery to slightly ease
bowel pain, leaving the dementia
untouched.

What shade of dementia? Does
Female believe that she's Maria Antoinette,
or that the government spies who shot
JFK have infiltrated the nursing home?
Does she contently wallow in life's reversal
back to damp sheets and feedings,
believing each nurse to be a kind aunt?
Does she envision vivid scenes—if only
someone knew to bring her paint and canvas!
Or perhaps she's wandered into blankness,
a creature of senses: warm, hungry, dry.
She's reduced to letters and numbers;
I'll never know, file her before B, Bailey:
aortic stenosis, failure of the heart.

FACTS

A well-planned trip abroad, the doctor thinks.
His map unfolds; he praises his wise self
for giving three whole days to visit Rome.
They reach the church where mute monks live and die.
The walls each hold a treasure chest of bones
like sacred shells. These strange embedded gifts
don't faze the brown-robed man who holds his thin
grey hand to take the small admission fee.

With pride the doctor rattles off the names
of bones: a rib, a skull, a clavicle,
teeth, patella, femurs, a coccyx here.
His lover drums her fingers on a rail.
Her eyes dart to the clouds beyond the door.

HEADING OFF DEMONS

Note to self to (maybe) head off demons
(this time): Crank the music,
let Patsy and Perry tug those
cliché strings. Have more orgasms
any way you can. Lose 20 pounds;
nothing as distracting as
a good obsession. Note:
do not obsess on person—you'll stalk.

Pop Prozac or what have you?

Erupt through mental sludge,
stay up late, thirty hour day
for the price of twenty-four.
Have more orgasms, stress relievers.
Buy stilettos and wear every
chance you get. Call Dr. Q.

Love: can't get too much.
Act out happiness or reasonable fascimile
of best recent photo. Lay vitamins
on sink by color—surprising
false sense of control gained
by organizing tiny things.
Damage control done by mascara wand,
waterproof of course.

Drop the gourmet cooking jag;
glorified housewifery earns praise,
is shat out tomorrow. Have more orgasms.
Eat out in fine places, ones with candles.
Wear those shoes.
Invite Dr. Q.

THE THERAPIST RECOMMENDS

that I go to Florida. He's teaching me
to differentiate between short and long

term goals, then follow a route
like breadcrumbs to a witch's house. He says

don't confuse the two, and whatever I do
omit emotion from any equation. This decision

to travel one last trip is short term; to skip
it is a figurative middle finger and that if you flip

someone the bird they will flip it right back.
I've lost interest in that tribe who treats me

politely of course preferring a young nurse
to heal wounded males. My therapist knows

about these things, and I muster what meager
trust I still can and Florida, here I come.

Don't forget to be happy or at least
smile, or pretend to, my therapist reminds me,

or else you'll be the only one in Disneyworld
wishing she was dead.

PAULA SERGI

HOME VISITS

No wonder I paused at their doorsteps,
measuring the distance between us:
my shining young skin, my white teeth, white shoes,
my crisp jacket, new job, fresh breath.
Before the knock I'd hesitate, checking their charts
for the wound where the pressure of time
had worn holes in their skins.

Most were near the end of their unpeeling,
shedding layers of memory and money.
On the other side of their doors, the acrid
ammonia of urine melted in their bedding,
their trousers and stockings. Drainage-soaked
gauzes trailed behind as they shuffled
to answer the bell.

I wrote *care* plans directing my visits,
mapping the way those wounds would heal,
from the outside in, and listed what I'd use
to fill them: ointments and creams,
plastic sheets like skin itself glued over
their oozing gaps. Orange-colored scrubs
or vinegar. Even sugar sprinkled on like faith.

With my little healer's tools I listened to the pressure
of blood against their vessels as their corpuscles tried
to escape. Catheters drained their amber urine

and plugged up and had to be plumbed. Urine bags
hung like handbags over walkers or bed rails.
I poured their pills into plastic cups, marking
time on calendars big as their kitchen tables.

But I was distracted: the corners of their homes,
the cobwebs and cuckoo clocks, veneered end tables,
scratched woodwork, what the windowsill
figurines could say. Sometimes I'd hear about
lovely mothers, the children they never saw again.
And when the hour was up, I'd shout
my instructions and leave.

It's not that I didn't want to touch them.
We had no idea, back then, about age
passing itself on. It's taken years
for me to recognize a skin that won't
bounce back, a stuttered gait on icy walks,
elusive words that hide behind
the floaters in my eyes. Once in a while

I'd see it when I washed their bony backs,
a used-up body about to lift off
with scapular wings. The glitter of dust motes
above their bird-like heads as they sat
by their windows watching me coming
and going, still lives of another kind. Above
little cloud-tufts of hair, haloes for the almost dead.

GARY YOUNG

I HAVE TO LOOK

I have to look, he said, and peeled away the bandages, unwinding them like a blood-soaked turban. I saw his reflection in the window. His neck was slashed; half his scalp had been sliced away. I wanted to feel sorry for him. I'd seen his leg. Somehow they'd removed the skin, and blood seeped through a layer of gauze and stained the sheets. His face hovered in the dark glass. You have a body, you should love it. That night an old woman lifted my legs from the bed, and set my feet in a little tub of warm water. This might help, she said. Honey, how does that feel? And while I tried to remember the last time I had cried, I cried.

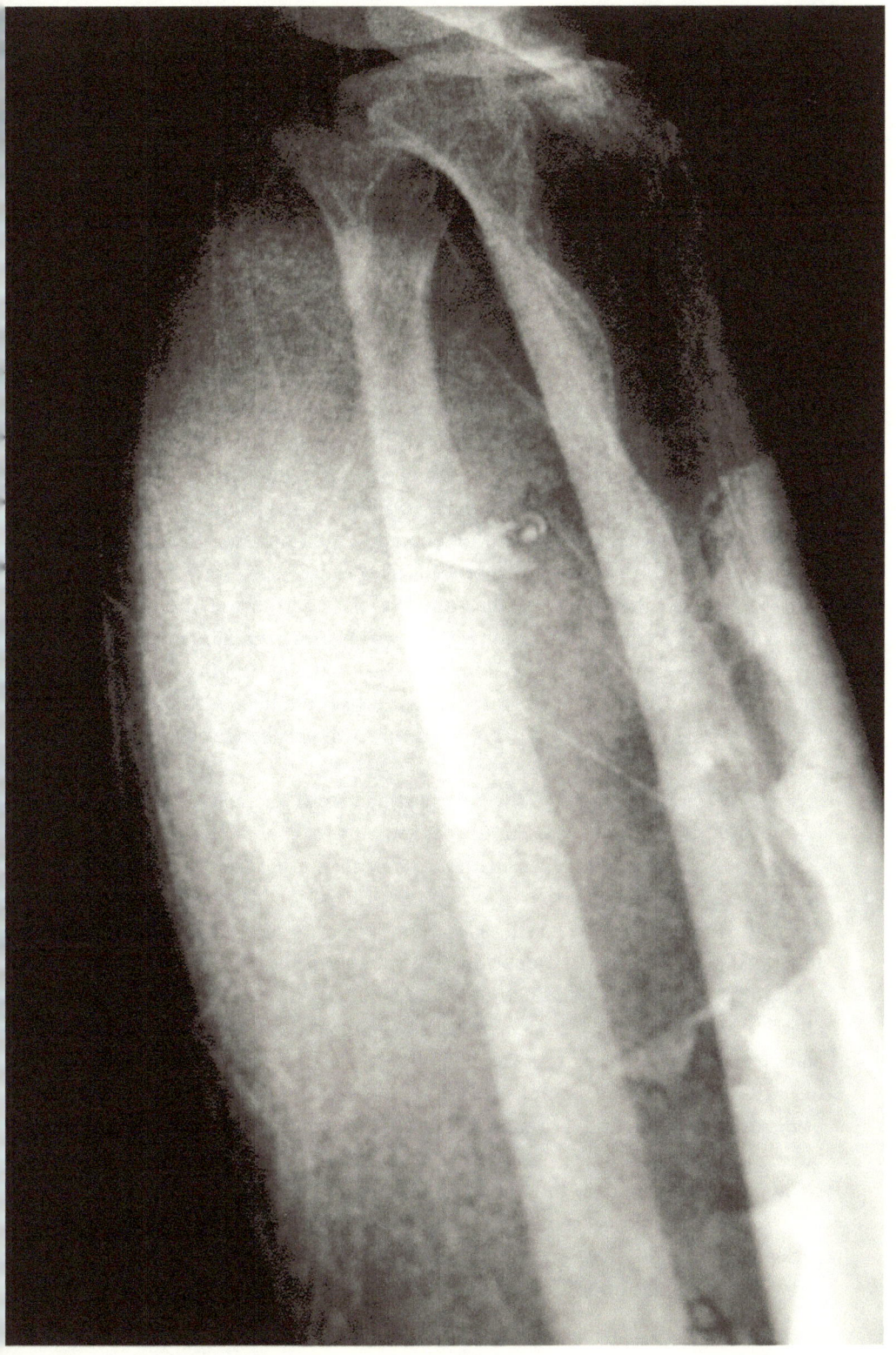

MARY ANN DiMOLA

EYE TO EYE

Most nurses wanted nothing to do with the burn unit. It was a messy, smelly, hot place and had all kinds of infection control garb that had to be donned. After every shift, not only were you sweaty and exhausted, but you had gold medal class "bad hair day" hair. In addition, the protocols for caring for burn patients were intense and took a long time to master. Recruits were hard to come by and nurses from other intensive care areas would not agree to "float" there. They were usually scared of the enormity of the technical and emotional challenges. Working there was not for the faint of heart or the vain. We were constantly looking for, no—actually begging—nurses to stay overtime or to come in early or on their days off to help with the patient load. For some reason, though, I was drawn to the challenge the burn unit offered.

When I think back to those early years I recall my focus on efficiency. I was quite determined to learn all there was to learn about burn patients, every aspect of treatment, every pathophysiological process, and every sharp edge of intensive care technology. When I left the patient's bedside at the end of a shift having finished everything—the monitoring, the IVs, the meds, the tube feedings, the bath, the debridement, the clean sheets, clean bandages, the splints, the messy creams, the respiratory care, the team planning, the charting and more—I felt I had a pretty good day. Even though most of those complex days were generally accompanied by missed lunches and the paucity of potty breaks, I felt accomplished. My chest swelled with pride when one of the doctors commented to me, "Oh good. You are here today. I am glad to have one of the best nurses taking care of this patient. He's really sick." The standards there were high but I was reaching them.

The emotional toll of working in a situation where most of the patients eventually died after many weeks or months of care, though, was more difficult to evaluate. To deal with the burden of many of the horrors we both witnessed and administered, many of us coped by distancing ourselves from our patients. We delivered care that was technically expert, we tried not to get too emotionally entangled, and we laughed, partied and jived each other all the time. We sought a release at the end of the day that often meant gathering at the local bar, frequently until the wee hours. It was at that time, in the wee hours, when I would finally get to sleep that the dreams usually started. Although I have never been able to discern with any degree of certainty whether my nighttime "visions" were actually dreams or nightmares, they were nonetheless very real and extremely vivid. Some were recurring. Some focused on the care I delivered to my patients or on my forgetting to give them some vital treatment or medication that could have saved their lives. Some focused on the patients themselves and their disfigurement and gruesome existence without a hand or a nose or eyelids. All of the dreams were disturbing, woke me up with a start, and left a lingering unsettled sensation the next morning.

It was on one of these mornings during this time of mixed sentiments, a strong sense of achieving technical excellence mixed with disturbing personal nighttime occurrences, that I had my first encounter with Stevie. Surprisingly, at seven years of age, he was the sage who helped me understand myself more deeply and in doing so, changed not only my nursing practice but my perspective about life in general. On the day we met, I was the "charge" nurse and running around the unit trying to keep a lid on the controlled chaos that was the burn unit norm.

Everything was in check until I heard it: rrrrnnnggg, rrrnnnggg, rrrnnnggg. The RED PHONE! Before even answering, I knew what it meant—we were getting an admission. I picked up the phone and learned a seven year old from a housefire was arriving in twenty minutes. I started to scramble. Move a patient from bed 20 to bed 4 so the seven year old could have a private room for the first day or two. Page the resident on call and do the impossible, find a nurse to take care of the admission. I started down the list of names and numbers as I had done so many times before, and once I had a live person on the other end of the phone line began my plea, "Hi, how are you? This is Mary Ann." As if a line in a practiced script, I received a premature "No, I don't want to come in!" before I could even ask, "We really need some help today, can you . . . ?" "No." Click. Occasionally, the more polite staff would make up a lame excuse to cover the fact that they just didn't want to work overtime. "Oh, I am so sorry. If I had known I would have certainly come in but I just made an appointment to have my nails done. Maybe next time." In rare cases, someone needed money for a trip she had been planning or some piece of furniture she wanted for her apartment and I would hear the golden words, "OK. I'll come in." The relief brought by those four simple words was immense. On this morning, though, no one was planning a vacation or needing a new sofa. No one was coming.

Before I could regroup, Stevie's stretcher came barreling through the doors with the EMTs at his side. By default, I would have to be his nurse and manage all my other duties that day. "Oh boy!" I thought to myself. "No lunch today." Little did I know what was in store for me and how my life would be changed by this staffing situation.

The first hours with Stevie were hectic and centered around assessing his degree of injury, getting him stabilized, and hooking him up to the many tubes and monitors required to care for him. Having worked there for several years, I knew that his chances of surviving the serious burn injury he had sustained were mixed. He had a large amount of his body surface area covered in third degree burns but he had neither facial involvement nor smoke inhalation injury, two factors in his favor. He was also a child, and children have the remarkable capacity to recover in ways that adults could not. He could actually get better and go home even if he couldn't walk out under his own steam. He had a chance to "make it" and I knew that I would do all that I could to help him become a survivor. Yet, I also knew too well that the future of his recovery was uncertain so I couldn't get too attached.

Stevie didn't communicate anything to us; but, there was so much going on that most likely we wouldn't have noticed him trying to get our attention. We were all too focused on his body and its needs. However, once the initial surge of activity at Stevie's bedside waned and the doctors, respiratory therapists, X-ray technicians and physical therapists were gone, I had some quiet time with Stevie. Standing by his bedside, he looked into my eyes directly and with them said, "I'm scared." I looked down at him and saw a fragile little boy with a round moon face and beautiful eyes. I can still feel his eyes. I can still see them and see into them. They were a cross between Carolina blue and cerulean, a translucent Caribbean shade unusual for eye color. And BIG! His eyes were wide as he searched my eyes, perhaps because my eyes were the only human part of me that allowed connection. My hair was enclosed in a blue shower-cap-like covering, my face covered by an isolation mask, my body covered in a blue gown over my scrubs, hands in latex gloves, and even blue covers hiding my shoes. The eye-to-eye contact may have been Stevie's only conduit to me. His eyes captured me. I stared straight back into them, connecting with him on a level that was unfamiliar to me. I could tell he really needed me.

He told me his needs with his piercing eyes and expressions that day when he couldn't speak because a tube was helping him breath. He needed me to connect with him, not just administer to him. He needed me to stay with him, keep him calm, allay his fears, and hold his hand. I can't explain why or how, but I believed I knew what he was telling me. I found myself answering his unspoken questions. "My name is Mary Ann. I am going to stay with you and take care of you. I will not leave you. You are going to be alright. I will help you get better." I held his hand. I took off my latex glove so he could feel my skin. He seemed calmed by my voice and my assurances. Soon, the morphine kicked in and Stevie fell into a restful sleep, his breaths paced by the cyclical paced puffs of the ventilator.

Over the next few days, Stevie and I became an item. Stevie did not allow "business as usual" nursing care from me. After the breathing tube came out and he was able to speak, he had lots of questions. "What is going to happen to me?" I reassured him that he was getting better every day (and he was). I joked with him, "You are so strong for a little boy. Do you lift weights? Eat Wheaties?" He would sometimes break into a big grin that seemed to make his eyes twinkle even more. Yet, the trials of the burn injury always interfered with those tender moments. Pain accompanied every treatment and sometimes worse were the temperature swings that occurred because his skin was gone. Shivering with his teeth chattering, he tried to let me know, "III'm sooo cccc-old." The warm blankets and heaters didn't seem to warm him. I was out of options having tried all my regular warming tricks.

What I wanted to do was get in the bed next to him and hold him tight so my body heat would melt the cold he felt so intensely. But, I knew I couldn't do that for a host of reasons. Suddenly, I remembered a self-hypnosis class I had taken a few years before where I learned to feed myself positive messages instead of the negative subconscious dispatches that somehow seep into our minds. These techniques had helped me improve my running stamina in the past. I wondered if a similar strategy could help Stevie.

"We're taking a trip!" I announced. His eyes said, "Are you crazy? I can't get out of this bed. And I'm freezing!" I explained to him that I wanted to take him on a journey in our minds; a journey that we would take together.

We embarked on our first adventure right there and then. We went to the beach in the summer, a Florida beach. Through still chattering teeth, he proclaimed, "I don't know what Florida is." So, I took his hand, and we connected eye to eye and I showed him Florida. We experienced the hot, so very hot, weather. We looked at palm trees that were perfectly still since there was absolutely no breeze in that hot climate. We burrowed our cold feet into the sand that had been warmed so thoroughly by the ever shining sun. We stared at the blue water that happened to be the color of Stevie's eyes. Slowly, the shivering stopped and Stevie's teeth became still. He closed his eyes and basked in the sun. "I like Florida," he said dreamily. He faded off to sleep.

　　We took similar trips to other places—Alaska when it was really hot in the tub room, carnivals when Stevie needed to have some fun, and the mountains when we needed to block out all the activity and noise in the unit. These trips, more than any traditional burn therapies, seemed to help that little boy cope with the hard reality of his life at that time.

　　As Stevie's nurse and friend, I started to experience nursing care as a soulful and holistic art. Technical competence would never have been enough to nurse and nurture Stevie. Almost in a role reversal, he instructed me about what he needed. "Why do you have to do that now?" he would ask when it was time for some procedure or other. I realized that the answer too often was that I needed to do it so my job would be easier, not necessarily because the timing was right for him. We started to alter the routines that, once examined, seemed very arbitrarily set. Together, we customized his care and even let a few things slide. We developed a shared understanding that allowed comfort to settle in for both of us, for Stevie in his bed and me in mine, surprisingly without burn unit nightmares disturbing me.

　　Stevie died suddenly one night, probably from a blood clot traveling in his small but suddenly septic body. I wasn't there. When I arrived the next morning to find his bed empty, tears welled up in my eyes and my throat began to tighten. For the first time, I cried because a patient had died. Yet he had become more than a patient. He was a friend and a mentor and I would miss that little boy who was so brave and scared at the same time. I mourned his fate and the unfairness of life.

　　Stevie hadn't quite finished his work in this world, though. He had a place to take me just as I had taken him on imagery trips every day. After he was gone, Stevie rejoined me on the quest that we had begun together in the weeks I cared for him—a journey of the soul. I felt myself searching for the essence of nursing that I had sought distance from in order to safeguard my own feelings. I learned through Stevie how to bring genuine comfort to my patients, not merely by injecting morphine or providing nutrition, but by really *being* with my patients when often they had no other source of comfort. Slowly, over the weeks that followed Stevie's death, I understood more and more how I could provide my patients with something they needed, maybe even more than my clinical skills—a human-to-human connection that took each of us, both nurse and patient, to a place with a soul where a different source of comfort could be found.

Months later while caring for an elderly woman named Angela, I realized that my time with her that night might be her last. Her death seemed imminent. She had no family, no visitors. Only me. Before Stevie finished with me I might have frantically tended to all the equipment and processes that we employ in intensive areas when death is near. I would have been satisfied to document every part of that endeavor and with technical aplomb maneuver the code that marked the end. Yet, I knew that something much more important was expected from me. Angela needed me to comfort her in her last hours. She needed me to wash her hair, to powder her so she smelled nice, to put lotion on her charred body for no reason other than gentle human touch, and to hold her hand so she wasn't alone. I was able to do these things for Angela because I wasn't alone either. Stevie was there urging me on.

Over the many years that have passed since Stevie looked into my soul, I have dreamed of him often in those nighttime burn unit visions. These messages, though, have become dreams rather than nightmares and are more settled and comfortable for me than in those early years. But Stevie did change more than the nature of those dreams, he altered my life and my perspective by changing my connections with others. For me, finding places of comfort through communion with others has become a way of interacting. The peace emanating from these encounters has greatly enriched my daily life and emphasized my many blessings. I have traveled with many friends and strangers over the years to find places of comfort and I lovingly thank Stevie for being my guide. After thirty years, those eyes, long since gone from all but my memory, still speak to me.

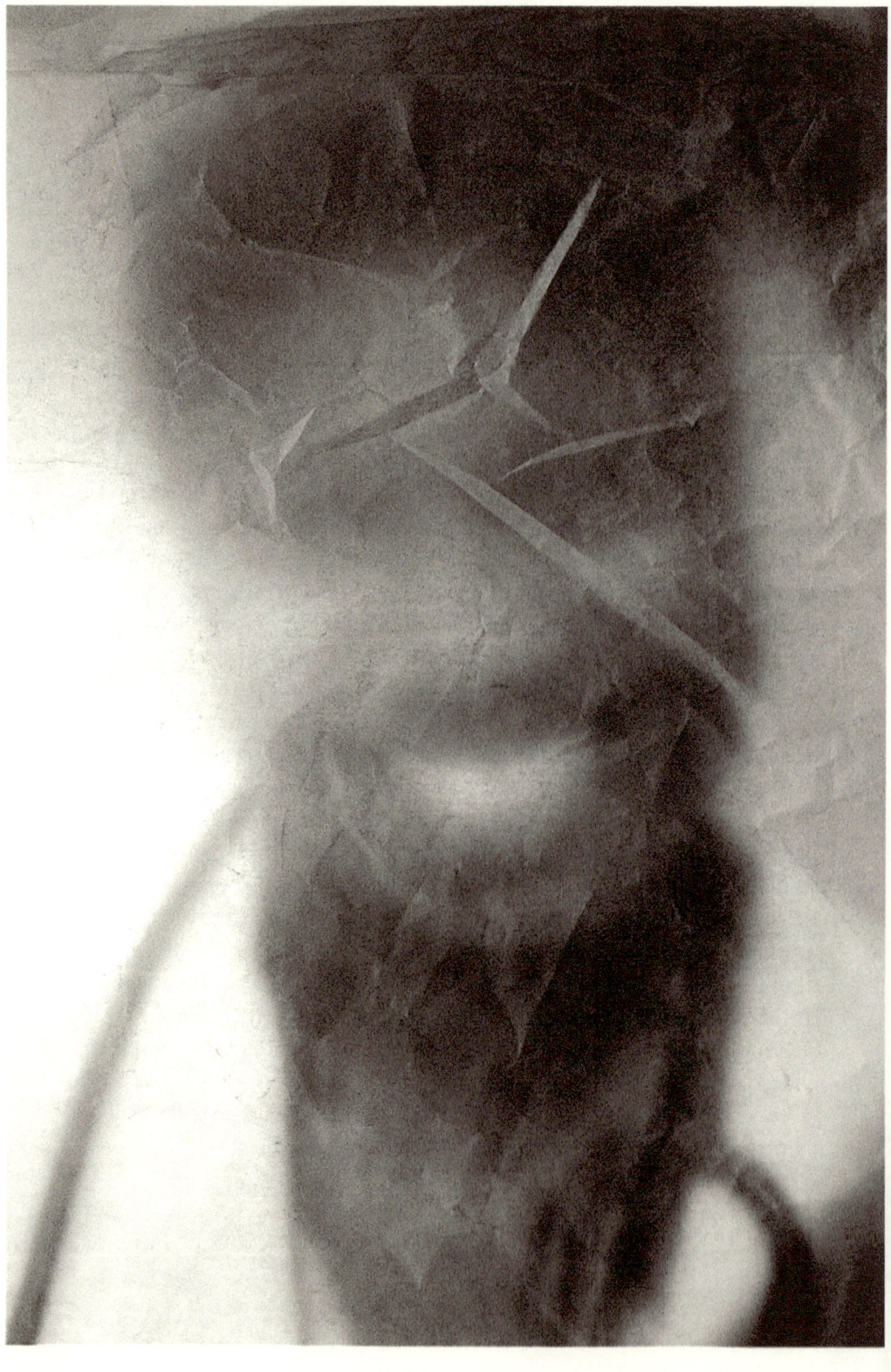

PATRICIA KETT

TO DIE WITH DIGNITY

The twenty-three year old
lies naked
unresponsive
smooth, black skin
flawless against white sheets.

Perfectly shaped designer breasts
thin waist
narrow hips
do not prepare the viewer
for the large penis, now dormant.

Nurses snicker as they call
each other
to view the "freak."
Another nurse
covers him with mercy.

He opens his eyes in a
blank stare
exhales loudly
dies in the dignity
he would make his own.

A GARDEN OF ROSES

They were married fifty-eight years
when Harry died.
After the funeral,
after the children left to go back to their lives,
after her grandsons left to go back to college,
after her friends stopped calling
Paula decided it was time.

She collected Harry's pills,
stopped taking hers for a week,
combined them in a bottle,
cleaned the house,
swallowed the pills
with a cup of green tea,
and waited for the white light,
for Harry.

There was a blinding white light,
and a crowd of people.
Someone bent over her.
Are you OK? Can you hear me?

Paula thought this can't be heaven,
the light is too bright, the voices too loud,
Did anyone get the daughter yet?

O no, she thought, don't call Maggie.
Shame washed over her,
not for her daughter
for herself, her failure, her, living.
Paula closed her eyes and wouldn't answer.
Even during the X-ray,
even during the IV insertion,
the nasal tube pumping out her stomach, and
the catheter being pushed into her bladder.

She allowed someone to cut off her
clothes, place an untied hospital gown over her,
transfer her to a stretcher.
Ignored the bumping through hallways,
a numbered transfer to a bed,
scrub-clad people
fussing, fussing,
Can't they leave me alone.

For two days doctors, nurses, and Maggie
called to her. She clamped her eyes and her
mouth tight. They spoke over her like
she wasn't there. If only it were true.
Harry, Harry where are you?
Then she heard someone singing.
A song. Their song. "If I Had My Way"
Paula opened her eyes. A nurse, singing to herself,
checking the IV, the monitors.
That song, how do you know that old song?

*It was my grandparents' favorite song,
it just came to me.*

Tears welled up in Paula's eyes.
the nurse reached for Paula's hand
and sat next to the bed.

Please sing it.

*If I had my way dear
forever there'd be, a garden of roses...*

Paula kept her eyes open
kept talking, crying, and in time,
returned to her garden of roses
where Harry forever would be.

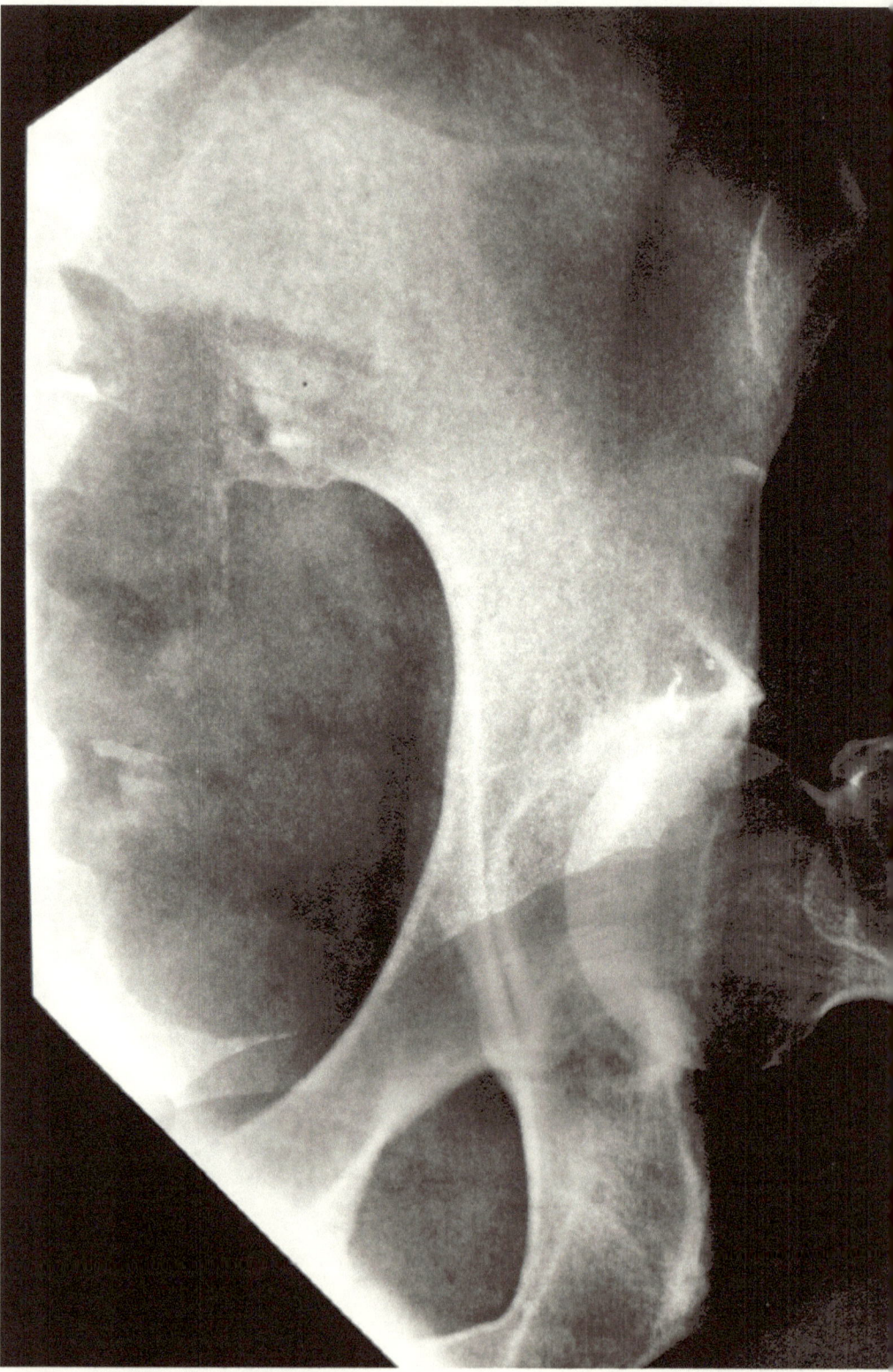

ANN J. BRADY

HE WAS 16

He was 16. Immobilized in a hospital bed, he had to wait for us. The sheets were rumpled, Hershey bar and M&M wrappers littered the tray table, bags of clear IV fluids swayed above him. His veins bulged in his forearms, the kind that made starting an IV easy. He had no tattoos, none that I saw, but he had the muscular body of a boxing champ and the vacant eyes of a coyote, averted each time I entered his room. He'd been shot, twice. And he sucked his thumb.

One bullet had ripped through his groin causing massive damage and swelling that required bilateral lower leg fasciotomies. The trauma surgeon ordered the protective dressings be changed once per shift. It took three of us to do it: one to hold his leg, another to cautiously unwind the gauze making sure the loose threads that adhered to the wound were carefully removed. A third poured saline over it and loosened any sloughed skin or debris. He stared out the window as we worked, intent on the mechanical equipment housed there. The hum of the outside machinery was constant, not the comfort of white noise but the low rumble like an oncoming train. It was a lousy room. He was in a lousy place. With his head turned away he sucked his thumb. I only saw the movement of the curled fist moving up and down, faster when the soiled dressing was removed, slower when the clean band of nubby gauze was applied. It was physically taxing for all of us. But it was emotionally difficult too because I was afraid of him. It wasn't the anxiety of adhering to strict isolation to protect the patient from my germs or me from his. I wasn't afraid of catching a disease from him. I was afraid of the parts of his life that might rub off on me, of what social contagion I might take home on my uniform. He sensed my discomfort, I was certain of that, so I labored to hide it from him, though in truth I was hiding it from myself. He worked his thumb the way my baby did when he was too tired to fight having his diaper changed and it was easier to turn his head and let me change him. I tried to remember my son when we changed the leg dressings, reminding myself that this sixteen year old wasn't really much older than my boy was. I was old enough to be his mother. I wanted to know the story of the shooting, thinking it might ease my fear. He was admitted with a pseudonym, not John Doe but John August, maybe because it was August and the ER couldn't come up with something clever. I didn't know if he was a victim or the perpetrator so I worried that another gang member might come by and finish the job. But I also was afraid that another gang member might come by and I'd have to figure out how to interact with him as well.

I'd never seen fasciotomies before, the layers of glistening pink muscle, the pale tendons and the ragged edges that pushed away from the swollen tissue. The sweet yeasty smell combined with a waft of cloying odor from the rim of scab. In my mind healing meant closed wounds and crusted suture lines, not the constant oozing of flayed calves. I spoke as I worked and directed the others, the echo of my voice a testament to my belief that if I sounded confident I would be confident. But it was impossible to pretend that his thumb sucking was not significant, to act like we didn't see what he was doing. I tried to bring him around with the few tricks I had in my nursing arsenal: humor, soothing tones, open-ended questions, but it was as if I wasn't there. He had blocked me out. I worried that I sounded patronizing and that was what made him turn away. I wasn't sure if he acted like he did because he was in the hospital and afraid, or if his behavior and lack of social skills were what caused him to be shot. He never spoke to me. He never answered my questions. He never made eye contact. I touched him but I couldn't reach him.

I am always learning from my patients. From some I learn a new nursing skill or technique; some teach me new life skills. He was one of those patients who did both. As I wrapped Kling over the wet 4x4's I wrapped him with parts of myself, the part that had to overcome my fear of him, the part that had to remind myself to be compassionate. Our lives touched each other. While I concentrated on being careful to re-wrap the legs correctly; cautious about where to start the continuous line of gauze—not too tight, not too loose, too dry or too wet, I also focused on acknowledging my feelings. What could I do to help him, what could I do to ease his fear of me? What part of me needed to change to care for him? The physicality of the dressing changes was as taxing as the mental challenge. I wanted my care of him to say something about me—that I had heroically conquered my apprehension, or at least quelled it, that I was open enough not to judge him. I thought my positive attitude would help me to reach him and he would see the effort I made. I thought if I did a good enough job that he would be grateful and one day when I walked in his room he would look up and thank me. I thought if I healed his wounds I could heal him inside too. None of that happened. He never shifted his attention from outside the window. My breakthrough came when I realized that even if I couldn't connect with him, couldn't make him see or be part of my brighter world that I had to care for him as if that would happen. His attitude didn't have to determine mine. Even though I was repelled by guns and violence and gangbangers set on killing each other, I could forget all of that and instead concentrate on providing the kind of care I wanted for my own child. I ignored the fact that a sixteen year old was sucking his thumb. I normalized it and blocked any negative comments or snickering about his thumb-sucking made by my co-workers and redirected them. "He's just a scared kid," I said. Even so, it was impossible to make believe it wasn't sadly pathetic. He had gotten to age sixteen without what he needed. As tough as he seemed to be he sought solace from the most primitive of stimuli.

Turns out part of him did rub off on me. He is with me each time I have a challenging patient, reminding me to examine my own prejudices, to take on my part of the relationship without blaming the difficult parts on the difficult patient. My experience with him made me search for the sixteen-year-old thumb-sucker, not just in my patients but in those I encounter outside of the hospital too. I learned that nursing isn't really about nurses at all, it is about patients. The cliché of meeting people where they are, in their place, is true.

It doesn't matter if he doesn't remember me, if I made no impression on him, if I didn't heal him inside. He made one on me by showing me that the turned away glance and the thumb were another way of coping. We all have our own thumbs, our own way of shielding ourselves from pain. He never spoke to me. I never heard his voice. Yet he reached me. He shook me up and I believe helped make me a better me.

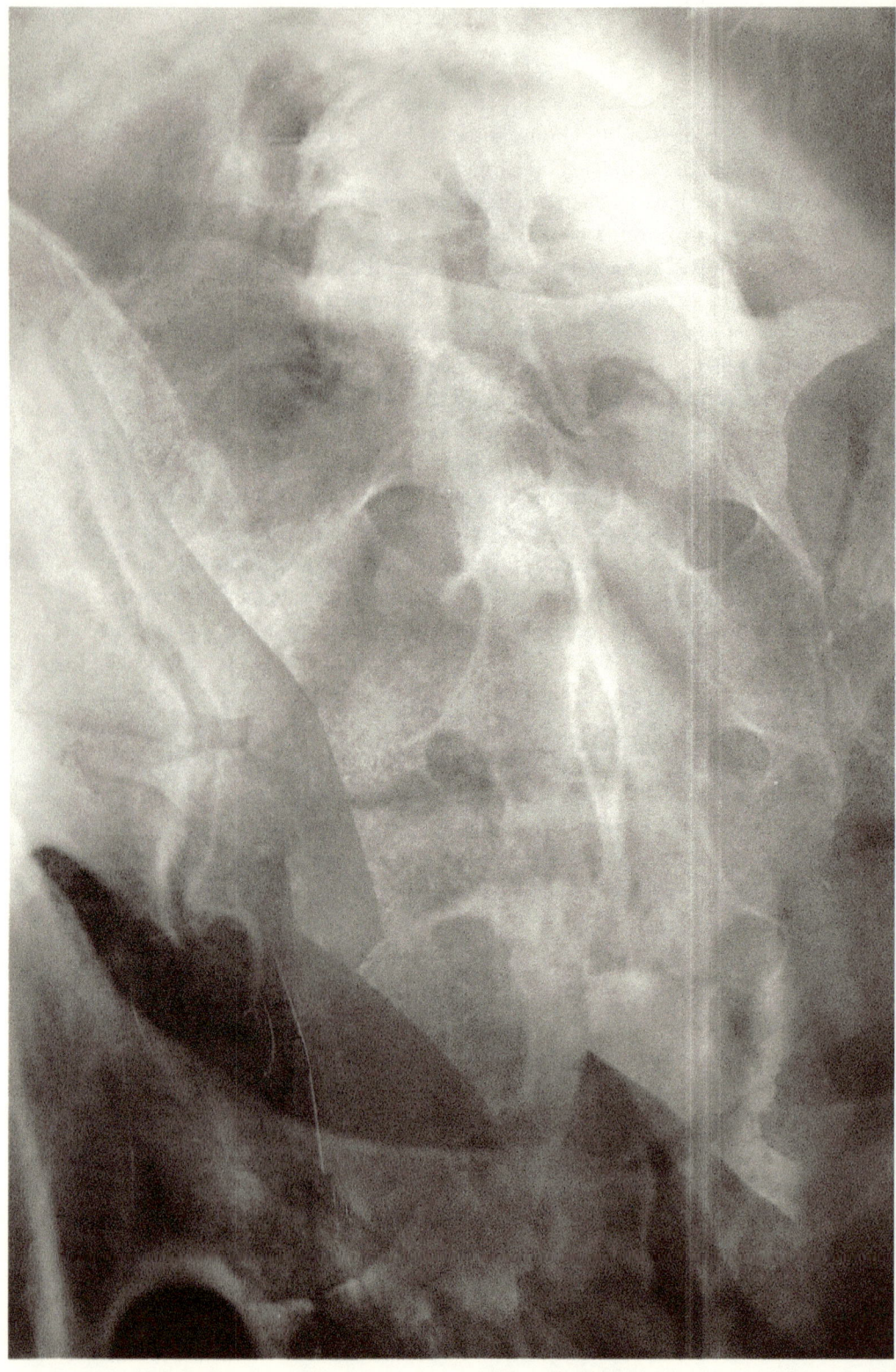

PHYLLIS A. LANGTON

DYING AT HOME

It happened after dinner on January 23, 2003, more than two years after my husband, George, diagnosed with ALS, was told he had six months to live. I helped him into our private elevator in our four-story townhouse to ride to the third floor to prepare him for bed. After closing the elevator doors and turning to smile at him, he looked at me with a fixed stare.

"Are you okay?" I asked.

"Yes, but I'm really tired."

As I moved around to be ready to open the elevator doors, the next sensation I felt was George falling on me, fast, and my knees crumbled as his dead weight pushed us to the floor. Knowing I had three seconds to open the two elevator doors before the lights turned off, I rolled out from under him gently placing his head on the floor. Grabbing the inside folded metal elevator door and shoving it back to the wall, I was able to pull down the handle to open the outside door.

Turning back I looked at his chalk-white face and realized he was a goner as he lay there gravely still. He was someplace else. Leaning down to his face to feel for air coming from his nose or mouth, I lay my fingers on his wrist for a pulse, while calling his name. He didn't answer. I slapped the side of his face. He didn't react. His rapid, thready pulse was barely perceptible.

I ran into the bedroom, grabbed a blanket to cover him and a pillow to put under his head, which I cuddled in my lap to be sure his airway was open. I rubbed his face, especially his forehead, which he particularly liked. I talked to him about the fun day we had and about our friends coming for dinner the next night to watch *Casablanca*, one of our old time favorites.

Yet, I felt the tension pulling on me to start doing CPR to get him breathing again. As a nurse, I should try to resuscitate him by compressing his chest, an important step in CPR. Instead, as his wife, I talked with him about this. Even though he didn't answer me, I felt he heard me.

"George, you look so peaceful and you're home. I'm keeping my promise to you. I won't resuscitate you."

When he didn't respond for more than five minutes, I pulled down the elevator phone and dialed the hospice nurse on call and explained the situation.

"Have you called 911?" she asked.

"No, and I don't intend to."

"Why not?"

My heart did something funny in my chest. "We've been in your program for over ten months because my husband wants a peaceful death at home. He signed a medical directive to have no CPR, no resuscitation, and no life-saving devices."

The line was silent. I added, "I promised him he would die peacefully at home with no trips to the emergency room." I wondered what would have happened to George if I had given into the omnipotence of the nurse. It would've been a terrible violation of the promises I made to him. I had to respect his wishes and signed directives as his trustee.

Finally, I told her, "By the way, I'm a registered nurse. If my husband doesn't regain consciousness, you have to come here to pronounce him dead. I need to get back to my husband." I felt dizzy as my stomach crawled up into my throat.

She agreed to come.

Returning to help George, I found him curled on his left side, barely squirming on the elevator floor trying to turn over. I kneeled down beside him. "George, can you hear me?" I asked. "This is Phyllis. Are you okay?"

I touched his right wrist to feel for his pulse. It was faint but steady.

He stopped moving and didn't answer for a couple of minutes.

"Do you want me to help you?" I asked.

Suddenly his eyes opened. He looked at me with glazed eyes with no sign of recognition. "Where am I?"

"George, this is Phyllis. You're home. Can you hear me?"

He answered, "I was on my way, but I forgot something."

Thrilled to hear his voice, I hugged him and worked to make him comfortable for a moment with his head in my lap.

"You forgot me." I answered.

"Oh, Phyllis, you're so silly. Nobody could forget you," he said, as his old, devilish grin crept up the sides of his face.

At that moment, I felt like smacking him, if I hadn't been so happy to hear his crazy, flyboy humor. The stubborn ole mule rider was doing his thing again.

"Where were you?" I said.

"On a trip. It was fun."

"I'm glad you had a good time. You scared the hell out of me."

"Sorry. Do I have to stay on the floor forever?"

Since he was warm and comfortable on the floor of the elevator, I decided to leave him there until our friends Harvey and Dianne arrived, shortly thereafter. They helped me move him into the bathroom because he needed to have a bowel movement.

George was holding court like a king when the hospice nurse arrived. She asked him, "What happened?"

"I tried to pat Phyllis on the fanny, but I missed and fell," he said.

His irreverent, self-deprecating humor didn't go over well with the young nurse. She said nothing as she continued to examine him, checking his blood pressure, pulse, and respirations, all of which had returned to normal. Since he fell on me, there were no signs of physical injury on him. No one asked about me.

Several days later when George joked about this story with some of our friends, several were indignant and shocked, showing their disdain for me by saying, "That's terrible. You should have called 911. He could have died in the elevator."

I wanted to say to them, "So what if he died? Why should I drag him to an emergency room to die when he wanted to die peacefully in his home with no resuscitation? Have you ever been to an emergency room at night? How long do you think you'd wait to see a doctor, if you ever saw one?" But I said nothing. They wouldn't understand.

Finally, I asked George to stop sharing this incident with our friends because I was tired of the criticisms from people who knew I was a nurse. They failed to understand why I didn't act to save my husband from dying, the worst possible outcome for anyone. Dying peacefully at home was still not an accepted choice, when there was so much technical medicine in the hospital to delay it. Death remains the enemy for many people. For us, George's victory would be that he was conscious when he died peacefully at home, relieved from the pain and suffering from ALS, but triumphant in the way he lived with it.

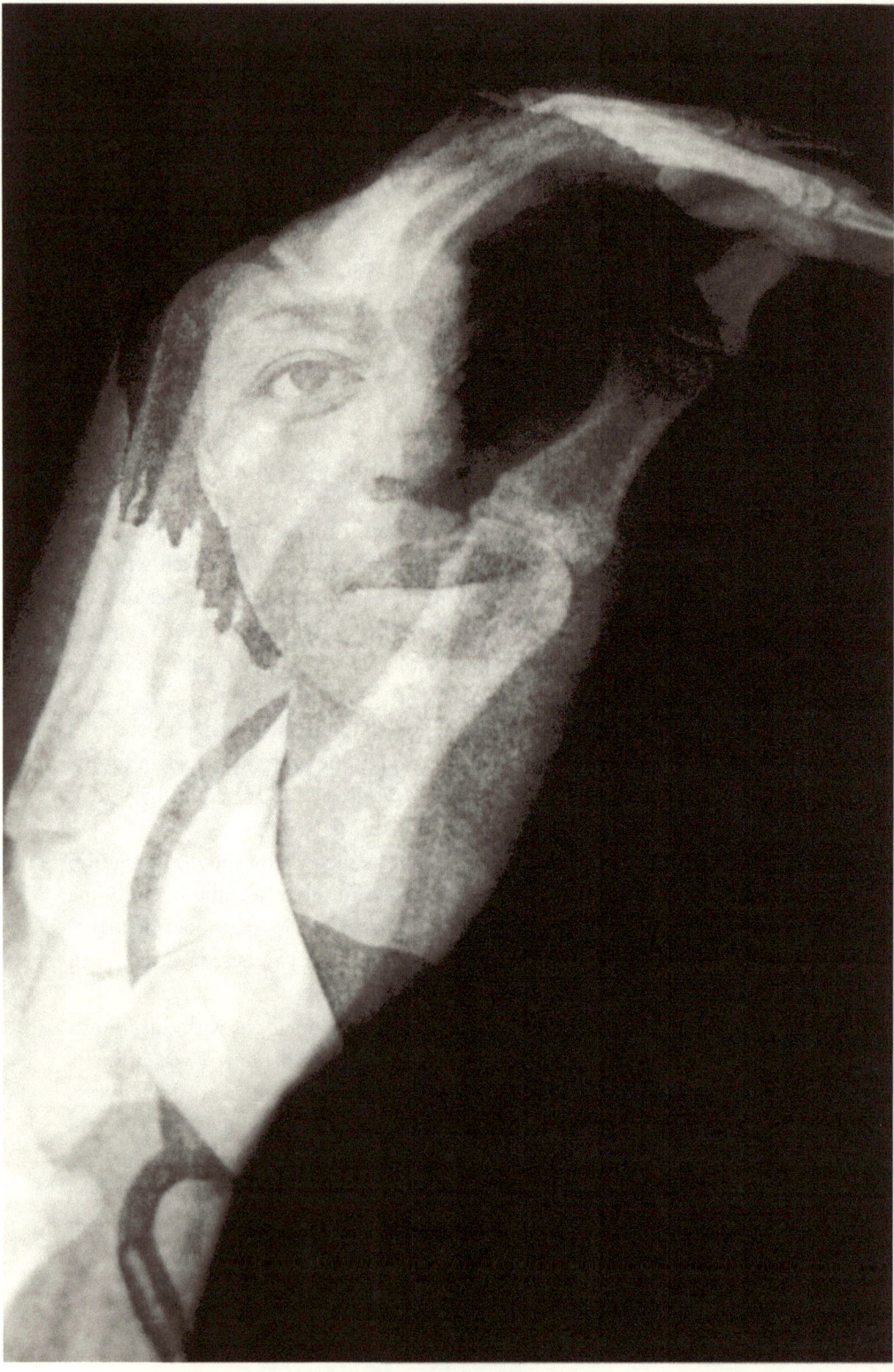

III
LONG-TERM RELATIONSHIPS

PATRICIA KETT

FOR BETTER OR WORSE

On their twenty-sixth anniversary,
a man and woman in a hospital room,
she upright in a chair, bald, abdomen swollen, eyes closed
he sprawled across the bed staring unblinking at her face.

He watches for a sign of pain. She moans.
He sits up and reaches for the call bell.
Waits. Waits. No response.
Kissing her he moves down the hall.

Ignored at the desk, he calls to the nurses
in a small room beyond where he stands.
"My wife's in pain."
"We need to count the narcotics, just a minute."

A minute is what part of twenty-six years?
How many parts love? How many parts pain?
They've loved, they've lost, now they wait.
She filled his needs, now he tries to fill hers.

"Nurse!"

NANCY J. BRANDWEIN

MY DOCTOR AND I

"It's not you, it's me," the man tells me, stroking my arm. It almost makes me laugh, because the man telling me this is not "breaking up" with me. He is my doctor, and he has been trying, without success to get an IV into my veins.

"But it is me," I say, in tears, "I'm the one with the bad veins."

"No it's not you, it's me. I hate that I'm hurting you like this."

Sometimes I think my doctor and I are like a long married couple. We've been together as long as my husband and I have been married, and our relationship has seen its share of near break-ups, rapprochements, and even celebratory moments.

Yet, the terms of this relationship are unlike any other. My doctor has an authority over and knowledge of me that I don't have of him. In his office I peer at the family photos, the marathon medals, the children's artwork— "We Love you Daddy"—trying to glean more about him. That he is a deeply religious Jew I can tell from the mezuzah on the doorpost of his office, the Hebrew words of Maimonides on his wall. When he comes in, his natty attire—lime green pants, designer ties—attests to a certain confidence and individualism. He, on the other hand, has just seen me naked and opens up a five-inch thick file detailing every aspect of my innards from the past fifteen years. The file also includes baby photos of my two children, an article I wrote, and a faxed letter that caused the first big rupture in our relationship.

I have Crohn's, a chronic intestinal disease that causes diarrhea, pain and fever. Four years ago, symptoms of my disease recurred a disturbingly short time after I had surgery to remove an obstructed portion of my intestines. My doctor prescribed a drug that he felt had great promise in stopping the constant diarrhea I was experiencing. That night I looked the drug up on the Internet and found it had been taken off the market by the FDA, that it was contraindicated for my disease and had the potential for very serious, though rare, side effects. My husband and I were shocked, and I immediately fired off a fax expressing my objections. My doctor called me back in a fury, pretty much saying, "How dare you??!!!" Yet, looking at what I wrote now, I see that it is not so much my questioning of his action that angered him, but the tone of my fax. What he heard was my voice beseeching him, "Why are you trying to harm me?" and I believe it was to this that he took such umbrage.

"First, do no harm." It is part of the Hippocratic oath to which doctors are supposed to adhere. Following this dictum, my doctor resisted giving me too many infusions of a drug that was one of my best hopes for remission but which has terrible possible side effects. It is what kept him from completing a colonoscopy for fear of perforating my gut. And it is what ultimately made him give up trying to find a vein and get the anesthesiologist next door to take over.

I think of how most marriages could benefit with the addition of "First, do no harm" to the wedding vows. My husband, Richard, and I never think of this warning as we launch into an emotional verbal assault. We don't wield hypodermic needles or razor-sharp scalpels, but our words have often been as damaging as any medical procedure gone awry.

However, wouldn't it be nice if doctors could bring to the doctor-patient relationship something that is common in marriage: apology? Fear of medical malpractice prevents most from saying "I'm sorry," but heartfelt apologies are the lubricants that keep marriages and deep friendships from cracking and eventually breaking. My doctor expressed remorse about episodes of obstruction I experienced after swallowing a diagnostic microchip the width of an AA battery when some of my intestinal strictures were narrower than a pencil. He also explained his rationale—it was the only way to visualize a tumor, something he was secretly worried about. Yet, he never simply said, "I'm sorry." In contrast, I have apologized to him on several occasions.

During one visit last year, no sooner had he walked in the examining room when I accused him of not taking the opinion of another GI seriously about the cause of certain unexplainable and disturbing symptoms I was experiencing. "You never told me it could be from my Crohn's disease!" I cried, implying that he was withholding information from me. He flared immediately into a rage, and brought up again "the fax" of four years ago. But what also had set things off, for me, was something that had nothing to do with my medical condition.

I had just published an essay, dealing with my disease, in a national publication. Excited and proud, I had told my doctor about the day it would appear, and he enthusiastically said he would look for it. For days after the essay's appearance, I kept hoping my doctor would call about the article, though I knew I'd see him soon. When he waved to me as he poked his head in the waiting room, hope surged. Again, nothing. During that messy shouting match, I suddenly said, like a wounded child, "And did you even read my article???" His face registered not only anger, but also actual hurt. "Nancy, not only did I read your article," he said, and he flipped open the giant file to show me the article clipped to the front, "but it was the very first thing I did that morning. I bought the paper and read it when I got my coffee, and I showed it to *everyone* in the office." Then, he flounced out of the office where I had to wait, uneasily, for him to come back and struggle to get an IV into my sclerotic veins.

I felt deep, blistering shame as I lay sobbing on the examining table, and at the same time, unjustly attacked. "How can we go on?" I wondered. Yet, when my doctor came back in, IV needle in hand, he asked, impatiently, "Why are you crying?"

"Do you still want to be my doctor?" I asked, my voice quavering.

"Of course," he said.

But then he put the ball squarely in my court, saying, "I think it's you that need to think about whether *you* still want *me* to be your doctor."

That night I spoke to Richard who had just been listening to Jerome Groopman discuss his new book, *How Doctors Think*, on NPR. According to Groopman doctors don't treat patients they dislike as well as they treat patients they like. "Listen," my husband told me, "You're not getting any better, and what if he doesn't like you? You could get a lot worse. Maybe it's time to switch doctors."

It was at this point—when Richard forced me to defend my decision to stay with my doctor—that I began thinking of our relationship as akin to marriage. "We've been through so much together," I told him. When I first started seeing my doctor, my husband and I were trying to conceive our first child, but I was in flare-up mode and despaired in my journal, "How will a baby ever take root in this thin husk of a body?" My doctor got me on a course of medicine that put me into remission, and it was to him that I went for the blood test when I suspected, but was too scared to hope, I might be pregnant. "Nancy, I have good news for you," his nasal, New York Jewish voice said on my message machine one bright January day. I replayed his phone message about a dozen times, dancing wildly around the living room in a stream of winter sunlight.

My doctor has ordered shipments of drugs from Canada for me—drugs not yet approved by the FDA, which, as he informed me during "the fax" contretemps, does not always work in the patient's best interests. He has given me infusions of the newest biologic medicines as soon as they came on the market. I have called him in the middle of the night, retching and in pain, and he has calmly told me what to do—and called me the next day to see how I fared. Once for five days in a row he came to my apartment on his way home from work to personally inject me with the steroids that would open the obstructed passages of my intestines.

"It would be like getting a divorce," I told Richard flatly, and then I used the words I play in my head during those inevitable bleak points in our marriage: "It's just a rough patch; we'll get through this."

So, I apologized, and while apology doesn't go two ways with us, forgiveness does. I think my doctor and I have forgiven each other "our trespasses" as it would say in his Hebrew prayer book. I have consciously become more trusting, less on the attack, and a better listener. My doctor's forgiveness of and commitment to me are more evident in his actions: he went to great lengths to get me into a promising stem cell study—the last ditch attempt at a medical solution that would keep a third surgery at bay. "Remember, you've never known what it's like to feel 'normal,'" he cautioned me, as I filled out the daily health diaries required to get into the drug study. He makes room for my sickness by acknowledging it, and that's no small thing. A patient with a chronic illness can be a great frustration to a doctor who is never really able to make them better.

On my birthday, for the second time during our fifteen years together, he called me up saying "Nancy, I have good news for you." I had been accepted into the study.

For the one month of the study's duration, I was in his office twice a week getting the time consuming treatments, my every reaction recorded by white-coated researchers. Once, while dozing off during an infusion, I had the vivid sense that my doctor was hovering over me saying the Shema, the most important prayer in Judaism. At the same time I felt my children's hands tugging on me from below the examining table, as if all three were trying to pull me into health. I woke feeling both blessed and befuddled. I took my dream as evidence of a deep concern for my well-being that went beyond any words my doctor could say.

Yet, as fervently as my doctor might have wished—for my sake—that the stem cells would seek out the inflamed areas of my intestines and heal them, he had his own ambitious reasons to hope for the study's success. Knowing that good results could help his star rise ever higher, upended, for once, our lopsided relationship. Not only did I want to be healed, but I also wanted to give him the gift of my health, to be one of those anonymous subjects who are said to go miraculously "into remission" when the study is written up in a medical journal.

However, it was not to be. While others went into remission, all I got from the study was free blood work and the knowledge that I would face another surgery. It was Christmas, and my doctor begged me to schedule surgery after the New Year. He put an X-ray of my gut up on the screen and rapped on the ulcerated passage with a pointer. "This. *This* is where you're bleeding, Nancy. You need to have it out."

Before I left his office that day, I told my doctor that our insurance would change in January and that he would no longer be "In Network." "I've filed for a 'continuation of care,'" I started to tell him, but my doctor put up his hand to interrupt me. "Nancy, I'm not leaving you now," he told me, reassuring me that whatever the corporate powers of managed care had in mind, he would continue to care for me as he always had.

JANE HERSCHLAG

FLOWERS FOR YOU BOB SIGMAN
In memory 9/9/95

who gave depth to my laugh
lifted the ache from my heart

You my friend taught me
how to make fist-words
and put a small kick in my step

Flowers for you who coaxed me
to sip the nectar of now
and reach into the cookie jar

Gentle doctor your voice
dissolved the ink-clot in my pen
Now it sings and cries

You dearest Bob
helped my man give me
flowers on an ordinary day

My garden rife with blooms
boasts buds year round
and thorns I've proudly grown

I bring you a varied bouquet
daffodil moon flower
morning glory and bleeding heart

CHANGE YOUR MIND
AND YOUR HAIR WILL STOP
FLYING OFF YOUR HEAD

said my husband
when I complained
I don't know how to uncoil

Trying to untangle the knots of my past
began the shedding of my hair
then my therapist shook
his index finger at me

Rather than run
to escape punish him elude my wrath
I stayed and stayed—
timidly shook my pinky at him

Dr. Hirsch shook his fist
though he repeatedly confessed
I know I've been out of control
I really want to work this through with you
You should confront me

No longer fooled by his granny cap
his ruffled collar sweet smile
I noticed his hairy knuckles
pointy teeth tenacious claws

I left expecting
long tresses again
and my intestines to stop churning

I'm still waiting

DEAR DOCTOR IRWIN

I've often admitted how devoid
of parenting I am. My mother-craving
exceeding my need for a father.
Neither are safe but a real mother
would not have studied her print dress.
She'd have danced even with a limp
to draw him from me. Her caress
would have coaxed my tears.

You seem a bit willing to be
mother and father but your
Victorian-reserve is not Mommy-Daddy.
Besides, protectors are swallowers or
rejectors. Orphanhood is preferable

to squashed, erased. I am grandly lucky with
peers of both sexes, loyal friends.
You say I'm unreceptive to parenting.
Of course. Wouldn't you be if
you were me? Perhaps I keep your
fathering at a cool distance,

keep you more peer, friend, latent lover, and
for moments mother, because fathers are
hammer and chisel. You ask, How can it be
that you need/want a mother and still have
not found her? I reply, I only want
a reality-based apron-mother

who doesn't wear blinders. I've never met
one, male or female. You ask,
Isn't that like a single woman claiming
there are no good men out there?
But people surround themselves with like-
types. I am too broken to befriend

a rounded, undented person.
I don't want to feel like a Martian.
All my friends are weather-beaten,
with smarts; they love nature and the arts.
Maybe when I'm seventy I'll connect
to a younger-generation-mother.

The older generation, blind-deaf-mutes,
hides in Fable's closet. You're the only
one I know not cloaked in myth. Except,
you insist you fall into the middle
range of female-ogling men. I've felt and seen

your glances at breasts, ass, legs. A thirsty
undressing, imbibing of me and others.
Average males view the same scenery
with less avarice. But since your hands
and words remain impeccable,

I'm annoyed but also glad
your eyes are cat-tongue-lappers. And after
reading you my poem, A Mother To Shade Me,

you sprouted leaves, shields against harshness.
But safer makes me hungrier.
Maybe I want the ultra-electra,

good-Daddy who fucks me with love.
It seems I have not grown beyond pre-
adolescence—I know you'll remain
my doctor and help me, as a real father,
to transfer my lusty-love to a more

suitable subject beyond these tabooed
walls. But as the hours pass
after today's reading, and your ample
shade, my groin calls for you more than ever.
I hate wanting what I cannot have.
This is precisely

what I hoped to avoid but since
uncorking my words, my cup runneth over.
I hope you too ache for me.
Just stay away from my ass
and my neck, and stay Doctor-protector-
father so I can become a real

grown up. I loved your question, Did reading
your erotic poem to me make you
feel powerful? It hadn't, but your question
implies I had power. That broadens my smile.
I like power, Doctor Irwin,
so I'll read this to you today.

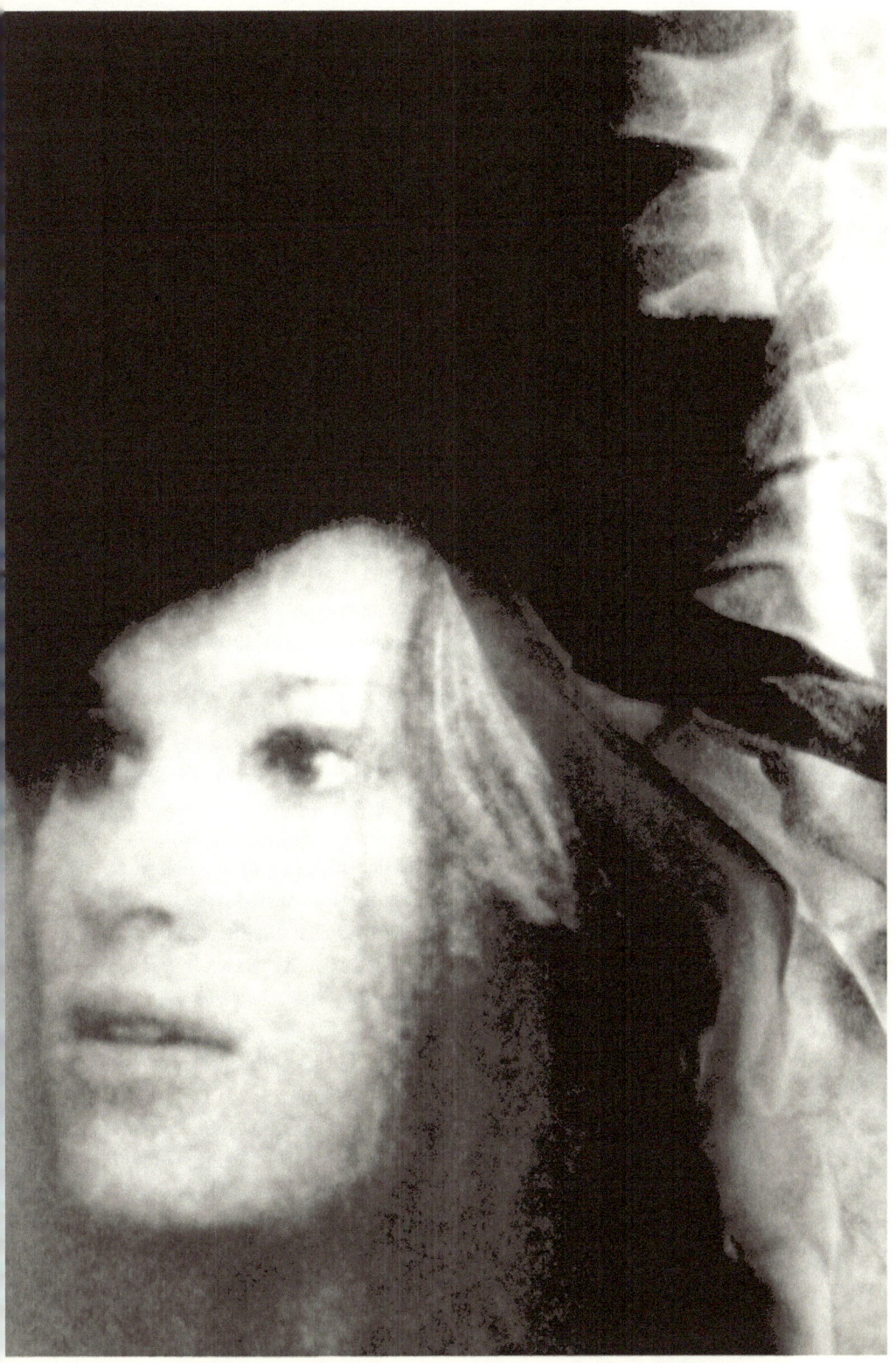

EVELYN SHARENOV

ANNIE

The first time I saw Annie she was in the middle of a handstand pushup against the wall outside her room. Balanced on her palms, her back and legs straight up, she pushed off without a sound. A cropped tee fell to her bra line, exposed the bone marimba of her ribs. Her tangle of auburn hair spilled to the floor and she had the translucent skin I associated with redheads; an appealing scatter of freckles dusted her nose. She looked more like a gangly teen than the twenty-five years I knew her to be.

"Hey," she called as I passed by. She rose on thin, sinewy arms without missing a beat.

"Hey yourself." I bent and smiled at her upside down face. She grinned.

"Could you help me? I need to shave my legs but someone has to watch me." She sniffed toward the clinical desk, "They're all too busy." She stopped her urgent pushups.

"I'll see how my morning looks and get back to you in a few minutes. You must be Annie." It was difficult to imagine her near death, but when I bent down to greet her I noted the black sutures that bit into the separated edges of flesh on her left wrist. Her self-inflicted wounds were almost healed, but I walked away with a sense of Annie's troubled life.

"You heard of me?"

"You bet." I had just spent an hour reading about her past. "I'll see you in a bit."

I'd been in this field two years, both on 3 East, a small community hospital on the east side of the Willamette River. The weight of Annie's hospital admissions and the severity of her illness challenged far more seasoned professionals. Her presence on 3 East was daunting. Her chart was seven inches thick—the clinical equivalent of hundreds of thousands of frequent flier miles—with information distilled from the records of her hospitalizations and outpatient treatment. It was hard to believe the upside-down in-person Annie could have burned as many bridges as hospital-chart Annie.

Joanie, a newly minted MSW, was at the clinical desk; she watched the monitors that illuminated all the dark corners and doors unseen from the station and that prevented assaults and elopements. She was new to 3 East, working her way out of the deep hole of college-loan poverty. We were a subset of a weekend team that included six therapists, five nurses, and five psychiatrists who rotated call. We had each other's backs in emergencies.

"Any reason I shouldn't help Annie shower and shave her legs?"

"Yeah," Joanie said. Apparently Alan, our second morning therapist, was busy leading a group. He had invited Annie and she declined. In report we discussed our strategy for working with Annie, particularly the need for consistency. Joanie and I were needed on the floor until Alan was free. Several patients were still asleep in bed or just waking up.

I checked my watch. Breakfast had come and gone while I'd gotten caught up in Annie's history. I worked back-to-back sixteen-hour shifts, Saturday and Sunday. It was Saturday morning, the start of my workweek.

Patients were admitted to 3 East in the acute phase of their illness, for assessment, stabilization and referral. Annie was admitted on Wednesday on a Notice of Mental Illness—a psychiatric hold for patients who posed a danger to themselves or others—with a diagnosis of borderline personality disorder. Because her illness had been well documented over its ten-year course, we knew what to expect, up to a point. Her overly bright greeting, the strenuous exercise, her mood of the moment could swiftly devolve into something dark and irrational.

She would manipulate staff, split us into enemy camps, hate us then love us—go from zero to sixty—in the time it took her heart to beat twice. She lived in a landscape of emotional extremes. She would rage at those who were supposed to love her, who perhaps did love her once, until it got too hard. She would rage equally at those who tried to hang onto her. We could expect her to try anything to fill the emptiness that—like an organ not visible on a CT scan but with an anatomical location vaguely near the human heart—came with her disorder.

Beyond genetics, we recognize people by their personality traits—the quirks and behaviors that differentiate us. A personality disorder developed over time, as a response to triggers like abuse or abandonment—real or perceived—and continued into adulthood if untreated.

Young women with Annie's diagnosis sometimes acted out in the form of suicidal gestures. BPD came with websites that catered to self-cutters and taught innovative methods of self-destruction. Annie shared creative nihilism the way best friends shared clothing and secrets.

When group ended, I found Annie. I turned up the hot water for her shower and brought her a cheap pink hospital-issue razor. She came equipped with a heavy white Turkish towel and her cosmetics kit, stuffed with miniature free-gift-with-purchase samples of expensive toiletries.

Delicate white scars road-mapped her flesh; intricate patterns crisscrossed her arms, legs, and stomach, trails of superficial cuts that dead-ended before reaching the generous blood supplies of her arteries and deep veins. I handed her the disposable razor.

"Not a pretty sight, is it?" she said.

"You look like my grandmother's lace curtains."

She giggled. The bathroom filled with steam, and I couldn't see her in the mirror. Uneasy, I moved closer to watch as she stroked the razor easily up her long legs.

"These razors are the pits. I never get it all."

When she arrived for lunch, she was meticulously made-up and neatly dressed in designer jeans and a bulky Aran-knit sweater, just a pretty young woman sitting down to lunch on a sunny afternoon. She wolfed down two helpings of salad with ranch dressing, three portions of Salisbury steak and gravy, mashed potatoes with butter and sour cream, and four styrofoam cups of ice cream for dessert.

When I walked past her room fifteen minutes later, I could hear her throwing up in her bathroom.

"Are you okay?" I interrupted the unmistakable gagging noise she made as she purged her lunch.

"Yeah," she called. "I'll be out in a minute."

Several stuffed animals rested on her pink satin pillowcases. She had taped photos to the wall above her bed. One photo in particular caught my eye. I leaned in to study it. Annie stood at the center of a group of people jammed together in tree-dappled sunshine. They posed for the camera, smiled and waved happily to an unseen audience. Annie looked healthy and plump.

When Annie emerged from the bathroom her lips were raw. She smelled of toothpaste and had changed into a hospital gown. She slumped down on her bed and clutched a shabby teddy bear.

I looked from her image in the photo to Annie in her bed.

"Who are these people?" I asked. "How old were you here?"

"Sixteen. My mother, my brother, my uncle, my cousin and my best friend."

I searched for clues in the photo. Nine years. What the hell had happened to her?

"Do I have to act out to get a shot? I just want to sleep now."

"I'll bring you something."

I injected a mild sedative. Now was not the time to discuss coping mechanisms. She skipped dinner and slept through the evening. Sometimes that's the best you can do for someone.

When I left the hospital that night through the sliding glass doors of the emergency room, I inhaled deeply. There was a disconnect between 3 East and the rest of the world. It was an occupational hazard. Inside, I often lost track of time. I was reminded it was Christmas when cards, gaily-wrapped gifts, and an artificial flame retardant tree decorated with soft ornaments appeared on 3 East.

Now it was the end of February, dreary and cold. Plumes of vapor billowed from my nose and mouth. It was a clear night, deep black with a dazzling array of stars and a sliver of bright white moon.

I pointed my car home. Christmas lights still lit houses and trees in Portland. I couldn't decide whether my neighbors were lazy, crazy or both; maybe they were depressed by our long gray winters or eccentrics who loved Christmas lights. Whatever their reason, that night I was grateful.

Although it's common, the medical profession does a dehumanizing disservice to patients when it defines them by diagnosis, particularly anyone diagnosed with a mental illness. Of course, the "Gall Bladder in Room 3" would probably be just fine, whereas the "Borderline in Room 7" was likely to be discharged with the same issues that brought her to the hospital in the first place. Strangely, patients defined themselves by their diagnoses as well. You were more likely to hear, "I'm a paranoid schizophrenic" than, "I'm a college student and sometimes I hear voices"—the already fragile psyche stigmatized by itself.

From her records I learned that Annie defiantly embraced her diagnosis. On a limited playing field, she took pride in being the best at something where few sought a trophy. It had its own perverse logic. She derived her identity from being 'a borderline' and saw herself as a teacher of other borderlines.

"I flunked DBT," she had bragged during intake. DBT—Dialectical Behavior Therapy—was the most effective treatment for someone as non-committal as Annie was to life's infinitive, 'to be.' It taught basic skills, skills needed to stay alive, like how and when to breathe, how to walk step-by-step past disaster.

Annie arrived on 3 East following several suicidal gestures, a smorgasbord of passive and aggressive attempts at self-annihilation. The serendipitous arrival of a friend usually thwarted her plan. This last time she upped the ante. She swallowed barbiturates, then passed a razor across her left wrist. When she changed her mind, she called 9-1-1 and left the phone line open as she spiraled down into unconsciousness.

Annie asked if she could talk to me.

"Sure. I have some time now."

She invited me into her room and collapsed onto her bed. I pulled a chair up close. Annie's features were distorted by crying and gaunt with weight loss. Her chart indicated she was down six pounds from a week ago. Her nightstand was a mess. Sticky remains of last night's juice smeared its surface. Used tissues dried into stiff white clots. An open composition notebook invited snooping. A cotton ball taped to the antecubital space of her left arm, from the morning's blood draw.

"How was your week?" I asked her.

"Just awful. If I can't get out of here, I don't know what I'll do."

Was that a threat? Why didn't she connect her suicide attempt with her hospitalization? Did she really imagine we would open the doors and let her out?

"Sounds like you feel pretty hopeless," I said. Although I really wanted to know about her week, my voice sounded thin and practiced, a bandaid on a hemorrhage. Annie spotted the insincerity and pounced.

"Don't talk to me like that," she yelled at me, then started to sob.

I felt like I'd been deservedly slapped. "Like what, Annie?"

"Like a nurse or therapist, whatever."

"I *am* a nurse. How do you want me to talk to you?"

"Like a friend."

"I care about you; I want to know what's going on; that's why I asked." How easily she walked over my carefully constructed boundaries. "I don't think you're ready for discharge, if that's what you're asking. What would you do if you got out of here tomorrow?"

She stopped crying. "They'd find me dead with a needle in my arm."

"That's kind of dramatic. And not likely to encourage me to advocate for your freedom."

"I'm nothing if not dramatic."

I laughed and she joined me.

"OK, you got me. So short of finding you dead with a needle in your arm, what do you want to do? What happens after here?"

"I want a life. Like everyone else. I deserve it."

"Swallowing pills and slashing your wrists doesn't say to me that you want a life," I pointed out. "It tells me you're ambivalent."

"Yeah, I get that. I want to write a book."

"It looks like you've already started." I indicated her scrawled notes.

"Like this." She pulled out a book she had tucked under her pillow and handed it to me.

It was a worn copy of *Girl Interrupted*, Susanna Kaysen's best-selling memoir of growing up with BPD. Corners of pages were tabbed down, doodles flamboyantly decorated the margins, passages that had special meaning for Annie were underlined in pencil. This book was part of the body of literature in this field. I flipped through it, read some of her notes.

"I'm her," she said.

"You're you. This book's already written. You have your own story to tell."

"Will you read it after I write it?"

"Of course. I'd like that."

"Co-ol," she said. She studied my face, momentarily hopeful.

I stood to go.

"Evelyn . . . "

"Yes?"

"Do you have to be so neutral?"

"Annie, you know the limits of our relationship. Maybe a shower and some fresh clothes, clean up your mess. It might help you feel . . . "

"Go to hell." There was something animal in her voice, growling, cold and hungry.

I kept walking. Neutral? When I thought of Annie I felt weary and sad. I wanted to grab her by the shoulders and shake some sense into her; definitely not neutral.

I was surprised when Annie made it to my transitions group in the afternoon. I had designed it for patients nearing discharge. It covered basics—your first steps after you walked out of the hospital into the daylight, where you were going and how you would get there; how you would fill your prescriptions. And more complex issues, like staying out of the hospital, and access to housing and healthcare—how to keep from falling through the cracks of the bureaucracy. I taught our most vulnerable citizens how to negotiate a draconian system.

Annie came up to me at the end.

"I liked your group. I learned something from it."

"Tell me."

"That it has nothing to do with me," she said. She smiled, turned and walked away from me.

When the doctor saw her on rounds, he spoke with her briefly, jotted some notes, and increased her Ativan, an anti-anxiety medication. Although his gaze held you long after you admitted you hated your mother, his approach was pleasantly straightforward. Many patients found this combination abrasive. He was not Annie's psychiatrist but he was well versed on her case—everyone who worked on 3 East was familiar with Annie's story.

We tweaked her medications. Until new and better medications came along, that was all we could do. Annie had been on anti-depressants, atypical antipsychotics, mood stabilizers, anti-anxiety medications and sedatives. They relieved some of her symptoms and temporarily improved her quality of life.

But there were no medications for the personality. One therapist, in complete frustration, had suggested that Annie needed a "personality transplant."

"Evelyn." Joanie's voice carried from Annie's room down the long hall to the community room. She was at Annie's side when I arrived. Annie was tangled in a mess of sheets and hospital gown. Her eyes rolled up in her head, her back arched and she thrashed uncontrollably, half off the bed. She was unresponsive and white froth turned blood-tinged when she bit her lip. It looked like a classic grand mal seizure. Annie experienced these after particularly violent episodes of purging. Alan got there just after me. We grabbed for her before she hit her head and carefully lowered her onto the floor.

It was over in an eternity of moments, and then Annie was still. Her blood pressure and pulse returned to normal. Her breathing was unlabored, but she was pale. I gave her low-flow oxygen through nasal prongs for a few minutes and notified the physician. An hour later, she was awake but sleepy. I sat in her room.

"What happens when I have a seizure?" she asked. Did her lips turn blue? Did she froth at the mouth? Did her eyes roll back in her head? Did her arms and legs jerk?

I thought about it.

"It's pretty scary looking," I answered.

I helped her clean up and change into flannel pajamas. I thought about neutrality and professional boundaries. Then I sat down with her and described her seizure, in detail.

She sat cross-legged on her bed. A tiny reading lamp clipped to her notebook cast a halo of warm light around her. When I left for the night, she was writing it all down.

We were worn down. *I* was worn down. I dreaded my long weekends locked onto 3 East with Annie. The staff met weekly for debriefings and diagnosed each other with compassion fatigue. We veered between giving up on her and belief that she was tough and would survive. We were horrified at our visceral responses of anger and dislike and surprised when our collective negative energy evaporated as she charmed us with a joke or smile, some token of affection.

She should have been out having fun with friends, attending college, enjoying a loving family. Instead she was spending her time with us, binging and purging, cutting, committing desperate acts of self-destruction. I compared her to Tinkerbell; Annie didn't stand a chance unless we believed in her.

She had a bad week. She was handcuffed and escorted by a Multnomah County sheriff's deputy to court, where she was civilly committed to 3 East for a period of six months. An older man who filled the role of lover, who was accustomed to the reciprocal use he and Annie made of each other, disappointed her by taking up with someone else. Her uncle didn't visit; her mother didn't call. She had been with us a month. A commitment would buy her—and us—some time.

One of the staff psychologists took her for a walk on the quiet street in front of the hospital, for some fresh air and a smoke. Annie ran toward the busy intersection and darted out into traffic. He ran after her and tackled her down; cars skidded and slammed on brakes around them.

That weekend I felt the prickly aftershocks of this incident. The staff was vigilant but gave her space. She was off 'constant.' I counted the number of times she paced the length of the ward—seventeen laps, a distance of one mile.

My stomach muscles hurt, braced against threat. We took turns walking past her room. I felt apprehension but not surprise when I heard the crash in Annie's room.

She stood on a chair with a fragment of a fluorescent light bulb that she'd broken out of the ceiling cage and slashed at her wrists. Blood dripped onto the floor. I grabbed towels to apply pressure while two others took her down from the chair. When we tried to pry the glass from her hands, she put the shards into her mouth and swallowed. Annie slithered and writhed across a floor that glittered with fragments of glass. Her mouth oozed blood as she bit at us.

"Code Green" echoed over the hospital speakers and trained staff arrived from all departments. The emergency room nurses were there when Annie lost consciousness and turned blue. We had minor cuts and bruises, and other deeper injuries that didn't show.

Closure is over-rated, and in our line of work it's elusive. Sometimes I read about a former patient in the newspaper—usually bad news, homicide or suicide or both. Or a photo of someone vaguely familiar poised on the Burnside Bridge. Not knowing was my way of holding on to hope.

Annie was referred to the state hospital, but did not meet their criteria for admission: her problem was behavioral, not psychosis. She was lucky; the state hospital was no place to get better.

Annie was discharged early, at the end of May into a run of good weather. She got better. She gained weight; she hadn't cut herself in a month; she discussed her behavior with seemingly mature insight. But I wasn't sure her improvement had anything to do with us.

In the next few months I'd hear rumors that Annie was or had been in our emergency department following yet another suicide attempt. I wanted to see her but I didn't want her back on 3 East. It was another hospital's turn.

A year later I found a note taped to the clinical desk inviting us to Annie's memorial service. There was a phone number if we wanted additional information. I didn't call.

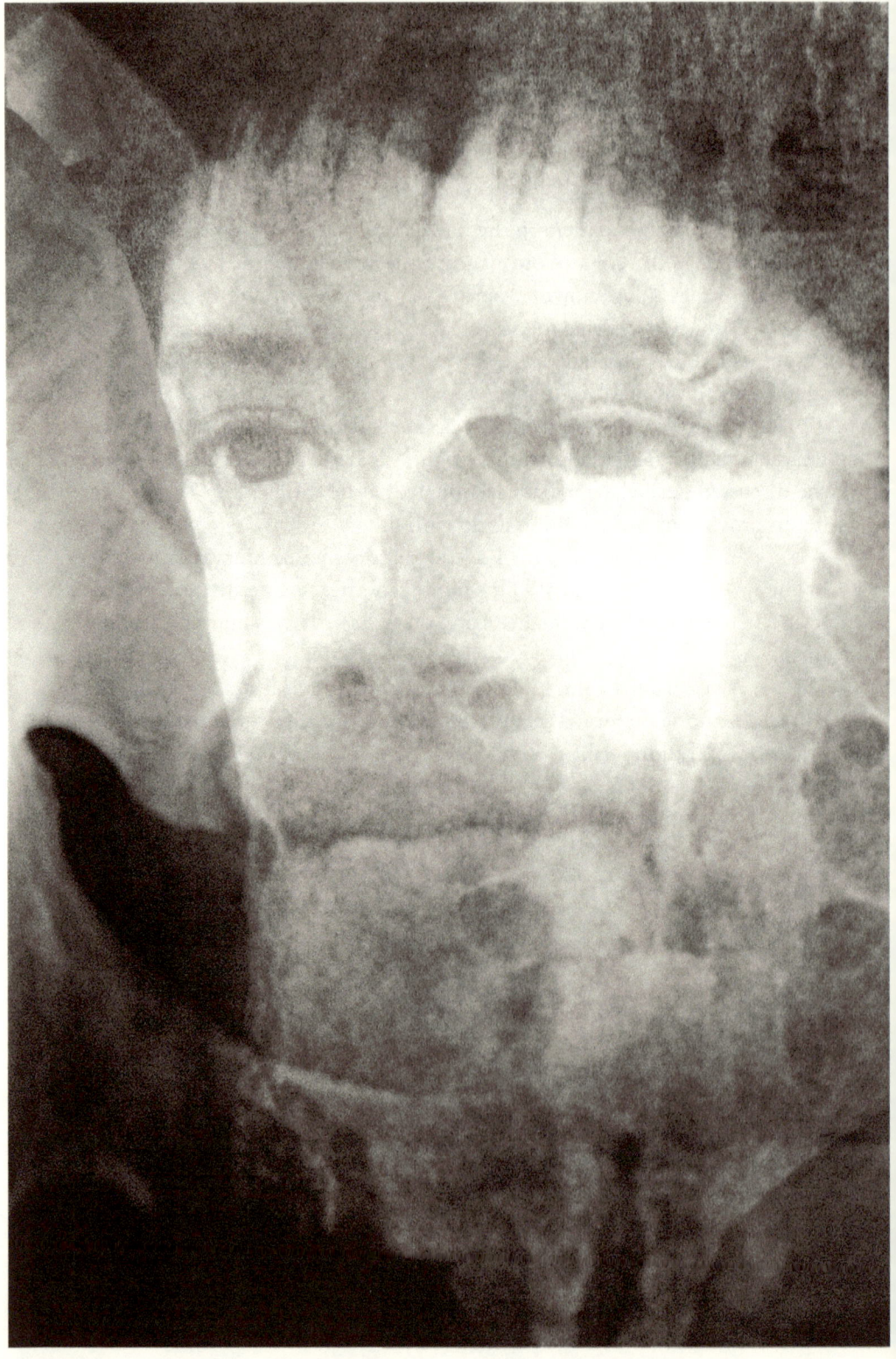

ZOË LOSADA

DAVIN'S ANGEL

I first met Dr. Pedro Del Nido in Boston's Children's Hospital, in the late morning of a Tuesday, at the end of a cold February 2008. My son, Davin, had had a catherization the day before in the same hospital. After the procedure, the doctor who was in charge of the cath, a wonderful doctor who had done at least five catherizations on Davin previously (I've lost count, I'm afraid) did not appear to give us the results. We waited and waited, spoke with the nurses and some residents who came around, all in a hurry to go somewhere else. Davin was discharged from the recovery room and sent to the hospital floor and, still, no report.

I had known, of course, that he was not well. The report from his checkup from the previous summer had been discouraging: a blunt confirmation of my observations. When my daughter and I had visited Vancouver with Davin before the check-up, we could see that he was having a hard time walking and was getting very tired. During the nights, I returned to my old habit of counting his breaths as he slept. Returning to Venezuela, we received the doctor's report full of complicated terms that basically meant that an operation to fix what was wrong with Davin's heart was virtually impossible, and that a transplant might be the only option left for him. We had come back to this hospital, as we had many times before, looking for help.

There are several pictures of Davin in our photo albums, taken when he was around three, lying on our bed, paler and more still than any child should be. He is dressed in striped red and grey sweater that match his grey corduroy overalls—an elegant outfit brought by his grandmother in one of her visits to our home in Venezuela—and his brown hair curls with a life of its own. I asked my husband, later, why he had taken so many of these pictures, and he answered that, at the time, he wasn't sure if he would see Davin again. Looking at these pictures, I feel again that cold desperation in my heart:

without my knowledge or consent, we had already started on a journey I hadn't planned for, and there was nothing I could do to protect this beloved, fragile child from the defects of his own heart.

This was the first of the many cases of severe respiratory infection he was to suffer for the next twenty years. His breathing was labored and fast, he barely responded to us, and he was hospitalized as soon as we took him later that day to the doctor's. And he came home again, resilient and strong. I'm not sure what caused these infections—it was never explained to me, but I imagine they had something to do with the edema in his lungs caused by pulmonary hypertension. This is a scary result of the backlog caused by the narrowing of the valves and aortic outflow track of the left side of his heart—a sort of chronic traffic jam.

Looking back, I realize that, at first, I did not see the many doctors and nurses that worked with us as people in a real sense—I saw them in relation to the help they gave Davin. I had no idea about their lives. Were they married? Did they have children? What were their hopes, their needs, their dreams? I did not ask these questions, maybe because I was not all that interested in the replies. Part of this was my own desperate search for a savior, for someone with all the answers, and part was the social structure of the hospital (maybe all hospitals). Doctors and nurses, and all the other people who worked in the hospital wore uniforms. Emotions seemed to be our exclusive domain, as the family, unmentionable and unacknowledged. The doctors and nurses I met had a totally different point of view about Davin and his illness than I did—I felt that, in a sense, Davin WAS his illness for them, and I was his Mom and my husband was his Dad (they would even say this in intensive care—"Bed so and so, Mom's coming back"). His sister wasn't even on the radar. I believed that they thought that Davin was a problem to be solved, and, what's more, I didn't care, as long as they helped him.

This point of view slowly changed as time went on. I realized that, for Davin's heart problems, there were no saviors, no final solution after which he would be able to live a healthy life until old age. I remember, eight years ago, waiting in a hospital room for Davin to reappear after yet another pacemaker implant, this one for a recalled pacemaker that was failing in some patients. (He had had to have another replacement the year before because one of the pacemaker wires was breaking, causing him to suddenly collapse after his heart skipped several beats.) One of the electro-cardiologists in charge of overseeing the pacemaker changes came into the room, visibly distressed.

"I just want to tell you," he said, "how sorry I am for all this. Wires breaking, pacemakers failing. I am so sorry for how much Davin and your family has suffered. One would have to be inhuman not to feel compassion." Given the nature of the technical problem, only the very sickest, most pacemaker-dependent patients had to undergo this procedure, another of many, many surgeries for them, and this poor man was in charge of all the details of the operations. I was taken aback—I realized in all the years I had spent in hospitals with doctors on this long journey, I had never heard anyone say anything quite so emotional, and I was not sure I liked it. Maybe what I needed for Davin were machines, or angels, or, at very least, a miracle.

And then we met Dr. Del Nido. The night before, late, we were finally given the dismal cath results by Davin's primary cardiologist. (I have learned over the years that no doctor ever likes to give bad news.) Davin's pulmonary hypertension was extremely high, and his heart was not working well, lowering significantly the amount of blood that it was pumping to his body: hence the tiredness, rapid breathing. This, of course, was not a new problem, but, for years, he had lived in the balance; the balloon catherizations had kept his valves open enough to allow his heart to pump enough blood for life, but there was still significant narrowing, and it was damaging the heart muscle. He had been well enough to live a relatively normal life, go to high school, act in plays, live to age twenty-three, go to college, but time was running out. His heart could not continue to function. The heart transplant I had been terrified of was not a possibility; the doctor carefully explained why pulmonary hypertension at the level that Davin had made this impossible. The next day, he said, forty cardiologists would meet with Dr. Del Nido and make the final decision. Could they operate and help him, or should he simply go home? We all knew enough to know what that meant. I left the room in despair.

The next morning, after the meeting, and after a visit from Davin's cardiologist, Dr. Del Nido appeared, a short, unassuming, calm man, who spoke perfect, unaccented, Spanish and English. He came alone, without the entourage that usually accompanies surgeons and explained that the operation would entail changing at least the mitral valve, and maybe the aortic valve, too. This was the operation that a surgeon had refused to do more than twelve years ago, discarding it as too risky (that's why Davin had had three balloon catherizations). It was a very difficult operation he told us, predicting two weeks in intensive care and a long recovery. Davin was an adult, and Davin decided: "Let's do this," he said.

And so, early the next afternoon, they took Davin away for his fourth open-heart surgery. These departures have a sort of ritual—the signing, the checking of documents, the endless parade of residents and nurses in this teaching hospital, the pill which always makes Davin laugh, and, finally, the anesthesiologists wheeling him, giggling, away, leaving us bereft and frightened. "Take care of him," I told Dr. del Nido, "bring him back." We went with my sister to the waiting room, a beautiful place full of light, with a view of the winter day, and we said prayers, and (no kidding), during a meditation, I saw the doctor, his hands lifted in the air, as if he had just sterilized them, light radiating from every finger.

Dr. Del Nido is not an angel, I am sure, and the operation he performed was not a miracle, but, rather, the result of years of practice as well as research by talented scientists and doctors, with the support and wisdom of many nurses and students. I know he has a family and a life, taxes, and a car. He is probably as grumpy and disagreeable as anyone else when he is tired and as fallible as anyone else in regards to areas that are not cardiac surgery. What he did for Davin was a very human intervention. And yet . . . when he came up to tell us, in a matter-of-fact way, after the operation that Davin's heart had responded very well after the operation, and that the problem with his heart had been the mitral valve, which he had replaced, and when, days later, Davin set off to practically jog around the ward, I.V. in hand ("The more exercise I do," he snarled, "the sooner I get out of this place") and when, a month later, for the first time in his life, he started a regular exercise routine in rehab, and when he raced with his sister and me on the beach in Australia this winter, and went hiking with us in the hills above the beach . . . this remarkable surgeon has been an angel for us.

I am aware now, as I write this, that this is not Davin's story, but mine. As he told me, when he was fifteen, in a rare bitterly communicative moment, one of the few times that he has spoken of the complex congenital heart disease he was born with, I will never understand what it is to be him.

From a purely physical point of view, he was totally right. I have never struggled for breath, never had tubes emerging from my body to get rid of excess liquid build-up after an operation, never endured overwhelming pain, and never been dependent on a pacemaker. I can imagine these experiences, because I have seen them all in his eyes, but I have not lived them. I can only tell my own stories.

As I cannot understand Davin, I do not think I will ever understand Dr. Pedro del Nido in any real sense. I try to imagine his life—he wakes up, brushes his teeth, drives to work, meets with distraught parents, repairs their child's heart, has lunch, meets with more distraught parents, operates on their child's heart, drives home, has dinner with his family, watches a ball game, and does the same thing the next day and the next and the next and the next, more than three hundred days a year—I cannot imagine who he is or what he feels, or how and why he does what he does. But I do know that I have no words, that there are no words, to thank him for Davin's life.

When Davin was fourteen months old, right before his first open-heart surgery, I sat with him in the Cardiology waiting room, listening to an eleven-year-old boy recite his medical history to the attending physician ("I was born with this, I had my first catherization at age such an such"). I remember having to leave, overwhelmed both by sadness for the boy and his mother and by fear for my own son. I had no idea about what lay ahead in the next twenty-three years—the open-heart surgeries, the balloon catherizations, the pacemaker dependence, the pacemaker failures, the wounds, the medications, the whirring machinery. And I had no idea of the feelings—the fear, the sadness, the heartbreak, the frustration, the anger, and, more than I could ever have imagined, the love. Would I have chosen this journey for Davin, for my daughter, for my husband, for me, for all the people who have loved Davin? No, never. But would I change anything about him and his miraculous life? Again, no. As a young mother, I grieved for the baseball or soccer player that he never would be, for the carefree childhood he would never have (with the contrariness that characterizes all children, I guess, he was a devoted sports fan and had no time for the many pursuits he could have developed: art, pottery, reading . . .), but now I am content to have Davin, alive, twenty-five years old, against all odds, in this world, as he is.

TIMOTHY FRANCIS URBAN

THE SWEET LIFE

By the time I met Dr. Mendelowitz, I'd spent months sitting in identical rooms while the doctors tried to figure it out. These were rooms with two chairs, and some random imitations of Rothko paintings on the wall, more like a business office instead of a safe haven. Every week I would sit across from a different therapist and discuss my ever shifting moods. Whenever I did finally say something to them, I'd look up and I'd find these strangers. They all had faces as blank as a new canvas, with nothing discernible behind their features.

These sessions continued, and nothing changed. The thoughts were still racing through my head. My paranoia would subside only when it was overtaken by bursts of anger. I acted 'normal' throughout the day, then someone would make some small remark and I'd get pissed. I'd lock myself in my room, grab a knife and start cutting myself. I felt relief, instead of pain. Suddenly the world seemed less brutal, along with the people in it. There was always this calm after the storm; maybe that was why I kept mutilating myself. It was as quick as breaking a twig in two, the existing tension creating a sudden snap. This happened every day. Then I'd leave my dorm room and meander over to the school's counseling center. My shadow would try to pull me back, but I managed to trudge along.

These sessions felt like a trap, and the doctors all said the same thing: I was depressed and bipolar. It was as elementary as that, they said, a simple diagnosis treatable with the right medication. But I was hesitant to begin something I could depend on for the rest of my life. I knew there were other alternatives. I thought learning about various religions would help, but this course ended when I couldn't bring myself to believe in anything. It just didn't *feel* right. I wanted to have faith, but something kept telling me this wasn't the right way. I fell into further despair, the darkness closing in on me. The horizon looked menacing and foreboding and I ultimately gave in to everything the psychiatrists said. I began taking Seroquil and it seemed like I was on the right track, but my existential questions didn't vanish, and my cutting didn't stop. Once I even went into the woods to be alone, much like an animal does when it senses its own death. I took a folding knife with me, and I sat on a log, staring off into nothingness.

It was then that I knew that the traditional form of counseling wasn't working for me. I needed to find an alternative form of treatment. I had heard of "Existential Psychotherapy" through books I had read. I decided to look it up online. Only one psychologist came up. His name was Edward Mendelowitz.

Our first meeting stands out in my mind vividly. He was a tall, slender man, with a tranquil face and a joyful disposition. His voice was soft, and peaceful. He asked me to come into his office. The first thing he said wasn't the typical, "So, what can I do for you?" All he said was, "Tell me about yourself."

I started talking about why I was there, and my past medical history. He interrupted, saying, "No, no, I asked you about yourself, not your past psychological history." He paused and looked at me, studying me, then said, "Tell me some of your interests, Timothy. What do you like?" So I did. We talked about all of the authors I was reading. He had read the same books I had. He knew all about Camus, Sartre, and Bukowski. He was relatable, quoting philosophers like Nietzsche and Rollo May. These quotes were intriguing and they piqued my interest, enabling the conversation to pick up. I told him about my struggles. One in particular was how I thought too much. Thought about things I tried conveying to my peers, who'd just stare at me like I was an idiot. All he said was, "I can understand why you feel isolated and full of despair. There's nothing wrong with your mind racing. That's something many psychologists will try to tell you, but haven't you ever thought that other people think too little?" I was dumbfounded. I'd never thought of it that way.

He asked me if I'd dispute my diagnosis as bipolar. I told him I didn't think I was bipolar. I didn't know what was wrong with me. This led to our discussion of an article titled, "Existential Depression." This type of depression comes on when a person isn't passionate about their life. They have a crisis over the meaning of their life, like Lester Burnham experienced in *American Beauty*. He couldn't find any meaning in his life so he virtually changed everything about it.

When I told Dr. Mendelowitz about this he nodded his head. He looked pensive, and then he said, "It's likely that you could be experiencing this. I won't really know until we've met more. There are a lot of things you *could* be experiencing."

The rest of that first session went by quickly. He asked me about my family history, but we were sidetracked and we ultimately began talking about our interests again. It was the first time I felt like I could let my guard down. A weight lifted from my shoulders.

When I left his office, I felt overjoyed and uplifted while I walked the streets of Boston. My gut was no longer churning. For the first time in a while I could look at my surroundings without a care in the world. I could just be. The experience was serene. I was a *tabula rasa* waiting to experience the world.

All week I anticipated my next visit. When it arrived I was brimming with energy and I had butterflies in my chest. The session started off like before. I talked about how I had stayed at a mental institution months before. It was a place where I was on lock-down, a place where freedom was a luxury. When I told him this, he asked, "Do you think you learned anything there?"

I told him that the whole place was this institution that cared more about money than about the individual patients. We were all in there for a reason, it didn't matter what that reason was. Everyone was treated the same. We were cattle. It was a prison where individuals were reduced to numbers.

He looked at me with that studying, inquisitive look. Then he talked about something Nietzsche discussed. He said Nietzsche described man as a herd, meaning we all conform to certain groups, but when someone moves away from the herd they're viewed as problematic. People see this as a threat, especially when it comes to mental illness. If the system can't place your "illness," psychologists sometimes revert to gimmicks for diagnoses.

In the institution I had no say over my life; it was in the hands of a psychologist who didn't know me. I was prescribed more Seroquil, as well as Ativan, and Celexa after seeing the hospital's psychologist for a mere ten minutes. Dr. Mendelowitz took this in. He was reassuring and understood my feelings of bitterness. His voice calmed me, it reassured, it never judged. When I saw him, it was like the outside world disappeared. He let me speak my mind. When I told him it was hard waiting for answers to my questions, he was there to give me advice. He was always sitting in his desk chair when we'd talk. He held a cup of tea, and everything was leisurely. He was an older man, but time had treated him well. His office was comforting because he had piles of books, books that I just wanted to search through and read, books that helped me see myself in a clearer light.

I began reading authors like Musil, Neitzsche, Heiddeger, Kafka. We'd sit and talk about them, the authors who tried explaining human existence. Dr. Mendelowitz was an old soul, the wise man everybody looked to for guidance. He knew all of these books, and could carry on a stimulating conversation about any of them.

One day he introduced me to the films of Federico Fellini. He told me to start with *8½*, a film I'd never heard of. I watched it after I left and was in awe. The movie was a mixture of reality and dreams: a neorealist piece. It displayed the struggles of human existence through poetic narrative. There was one quote that I'll never forget, "Accept me as I am, not as I'd like to be." A light began to swell inside me. I was always that person standing on the wrong side of the bridge. The idea of being normal was appealing to me, but now I could see it was okay to be different.

Dr. Mendelowitz introduced me to a whole new world. He helped me regain control. When I feel the impulse to cut, I go to a quiet place and close my eyes. I think about all the texts I've read and what they've taught me. My head becomes clear. I know Dr. Mendelowitz won't always be there for me, but I'll always be here for myself. Someday my mentor will fade from my sight. Everything is finite, and nothing lasts forever. We will always struggle, and I know I will struggle in the future, but I can never let the darkness get in the way of *La Dolce Vita*: The Sweet Life.

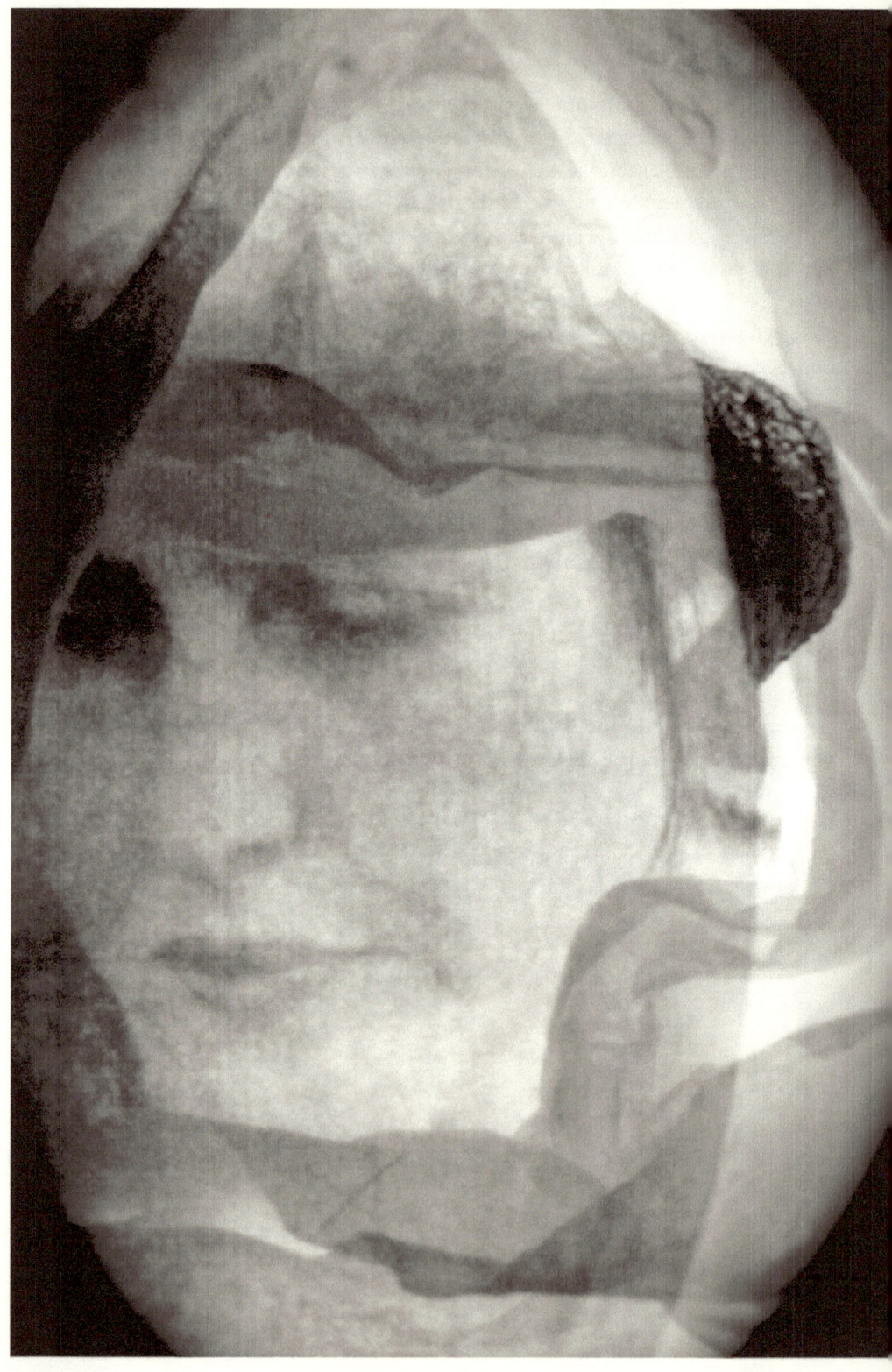

IV
DEFINING EXPERIENCE:
THE POWER OF WORDS

PAUL HOSTOVSKY

OTHER PEOPLE'S PAIN

My dentist told me when I was ten
that some people don't even need Novocain—
different thresholds for different
ten year olds. This was in Irvington
New Jersey in 1968, right after
I thrashed and bucked in his chair
which reared up on its hind legs
when the Novocain didn't work, and the pain
for which there were no words in the whole
world wouldn't fit inside my head.
And I started to cry.
I still can't get my head around
other people's pain being any
different from mine. I have yet to meet
someone who can fit the pain of the world
into the tiny cavity of a deciduous tooth
without a little Novocain. That being said,
it's hard to imagine the pain of all the people
in pain all over the world. I can only
really imagine the pain of one person—
because I am only one person—and even that
is made complicated by what a dentist said
about thresholds when I was ten. I suspect
I'm a wimp. I suspect another person—
a better person or a stronger person or just
a person with a higher threshold for pain—
wouldn't crumple under the pain that is my pain
if it were theirs. But if it *were* theirs,
and if they were one of the tribe that needs
Novocain, and if the Novocain didn't work,
I could imagine that. I could have compassion.

MATTHEW B. SMITH

THE GIFT

Monday was the day I performed procedures. I had eight cases scheduled at the hospital. Cathy had come for a colonoscopy as part of an evaluation of her anemia. She seemed a bit nervous as I greeted her, not making eye contact. This was not the same smiling, talkative woman I remembered from the consultation at my office the previous week. I held her hand and reassured her about the procedure. By the time we were ready to start she appeared visibly more relaxed.

During her colonoscopy I found a polyp. This is a growth in the colon that might grow into a colon cancer. It needed to be removed but it was located adjacent to the appendix. This is a delicate part of the colon with a thin wall. Removing a polyp in this location carries a higher risk of causing a bowel perforation. After I had carefully removed the polyp and she had woken from sedation I explained to Cathy and her husband that a polyp had been removed but that I had concerns about her risk of complications. I advised her not to eat any solid food for the rest of the day and to call me if she had any pain.

That evening she called. She said that at around four o'clock she developed a sudden pain in the lower right side of her abdomen, near where the appendix is located. My face went cold and my gut clenched. I thought "Oh no, she's perforated!" This is the dread of every physician. Although we accept that there is the trade off of a small risk of complication from any procedure in order to help a patient, when something we've done results in harm to someone it is devastating.

I met Cathy at the hospital that evening. Initial X-rays did not show a perforation but she was quite tender by then and had developed a fever. I spoke with her at length, telling her I was still concerned that she might be developing a perforation and that I wanted to treat her with antibiotics and order further testing including a CAT scan. Many patients would be angry, even accusatory after such an event but Cindy was not and I was grateful for this. She and her family had many questions. I tried to answer them all as best as I could. When I left the hospital that night I was emotionally and physically exhausted but I didn't sleep well. I lay awake replaying the colonoscopy in my head, trying to think of what I might have done differently.

The next day brought good news. The CAT scan showed no perforation. Moreover, her fever was gone and her pain had improved. I shared the good report with her. Her face brightened and I saw the same bubbly, smiling person I remembered from our initial office visit. We talked about what had probably happened: that the cautery had weakened the wall of the colon without causing a complete perforation. After a lull in the conversation she looked away. When she looked back directly at me her smile had faded. "I need to tell you something" she said firmly. "When I first met you I did not like you."

I sat there speechless. This is not an easy thing to hear, especially in a profession where relationships are so important. In the silence that followed she waited and then continued. "When I came to see you in your office you seemed to be in a hurry. You spent only a few minutes talking to me and examining me, and after discussing the procedure you recommended, you were out the door to see the next patient."

I looked at her, stunned. Had I really been that thoughtless? Had I rushed her? Had I ignored a worried look that might have alerted me to questions or fears that I hadn't let her express?

She went on. "But then you came to see me in the hospital. You sat by my bed and explained things to me. You took the time and I could see that you cared. That's when I started to like you."

I held back the tears. Yes, I did care. But I felt terrible about how I had treated her in my office.

That evening I thought about the day of her office visit. It had been a very busy day. Sick patients had to be added to an already full clinic schedule. These patients' problems took time to evaluate and I had gotten farther and farther behind. I was grateful that Cathy had such a simple problem. Anemia with relatively few symptoms was a bread-and-butter case. I could handle this in a short while and catch up on my other waiting patients. Cathy was right. I had rushed her through to get to the next patient. Now I thought of her sitting in my office after I'd left. What questions had gone unanswered? What fears left unvoiced? Issues that had become routine and rote to me were neither routine nor familiar to her. As I pondered our initial encounter from her perspective I began to wonder if in the midst of a busy practice I had somehow lost something.

I thought back to medical school and those first tentative contacts with 'real patients.' The science, the technology, the diseases fascinated me. But the interaction with people, the chance to help someone in pain, the privilege of sharing an intimacy necessitated by a patient's state of vulnerability and the opportunity to cherish and respect this responsibility, this is what made me love medicine. I have been profoundly lucky to have a job that can give as much as it asks of me.

But Cathy's comments were humbling. I wondered how often I had done this to others with 'routine' problems. How many had felt as Cathy had but hadn't bothered to tell me? I was struck by the courage it must have taken to say what she had said to me. How much easier would it have been just to have said nothing?

I went to see her the next day at the hospital. "You're doing well," I told her. "We can discharge you later today." I paused. "About what you said to me yesterday . . ." Her eyes dropped. I could tell she felt badly. "Thank you," I said. "You have given me a precious gift. You've helped me to remember why I chose to go into medicine. I'm grateful that you are the kind of person that you are and that you thought enough of me to tell me how I had treated you. It must not have been easy."

"No," she laughed, "it wasn't."

Clinics after that day were different. Patients with problems that I had seen a thousand times, I now saw through the eyes of someone for whom it was a new and possibly scary concern. I felt the newness of that special connection with patients that I remembered from medical school. Clinic was not a burden to complete, but a series of personal interactions I was privileged to be a part of. Of course, there are still good days and bad ones, easy days and days so busy my head spins. But now when I'm busy I take a deep breath before entering the next room and remember what Cathy taught me. And I love what I do all the more.

Thank you Cathy.

MARIETTE LANDRY

PATIENT EDUCATION

Back then I wasn't patient
or patient—just a visitor
in intensive care,
my aunt dead on
one side after a midnight
stroke, still happy to see me,
still giving advice, still
fighting for the last word.

She said, *he's no good.*
She meant my no-good love, the last
in a string of no-good loves
and the one I left, hours later,
speechless, because I saw it was time
to grow into the life I was
given, where waiting is an art,
a lesson in failure and forgiveness,

like anything else worth knowing,
since time is always behind you,
and words always matter.

TALKING

At the other end of the exam table—when
you least feel like talking—the doctor went on
about the great run he had last Sunday in the 5K, how
he'd beaten his personal best, what a great feeling that was,
and wow, he said, you have a beautiful cervix. What
I wanted to say—feeling heat in my cheeks
from this strange symbiosis of indignity and
pride, from the megawatt lamp set on high
beneath the flowered sheet over my knees and
under which all of his talking took place—was
talk to the hand, or save it for later, or just . . . *really?*
But given the awkward position he'd put me in,
I took a deep breath, looked up at the ceiling, said thanks.

CLAUDIA VAN GERVEN

"AS BENIGN AS BREAST TISSUE CAN BE,"

the young surgeon says
so matter-of-factly, I wonder
at the treachery of breast tissue,
how it must tangle itself uninvited
in a man's life, the first frantic search
for the fragrant nipple, the tell-tale
taste of sweet blue milk,
how he rose to it happy as a dolphin
frisking in rich, warm waters, where
he could drift away safe
on those steady currents and how suddenly
he was denied without a word
for betrayal, left
with cold plastic cup, tacky
rubber pacifier, his own
juiceless thumb

and none of this he can remember
or wants to, the girls in first grade
mercifully without such devious tissue
and he learns he is better, stronger
can hit the ball, can hit them and run
faster than the happy dolphin, faster than
the fragrant rivers of his wordless dreams

when all unsuspecting in Junior High
they assert themselves again, randomly
in the hallways, in forbidden magazines
are foreign, exotic, somehow
connected with his manhood, with the new
rise and fall of his dreams

and for the rest of his days
breast tissue will plaster itself
across his horizon, leap off
of billboards, caterwaul from his TV,
wrap itself around all his pleasures
liquor bottles, the Lotus Esprit,
complicate everything, self-willed
and elusive, unaccountably cruel, defying
even his medical skills,
mutating wildly, hiding
from his X-ray machine, tatting
out cancers to confound his blade, hording
everything, his toxins, his wastes
his son's stories of
a happy sea, a white island and a fish
that would never be caught.

CAROLYN McAULIFFE

SHORT BUS

Terbutaline, Nifedipine, Indomethacin, Glutocorticoids. My two months and change of bed rest opened me up to a whole new lexicon—a pharma-lexicon to be exact. At twenty-five and a half weeks following my unborn baby's first attempt to prematurely exit my womb, my newly diagnosed precarious condition of uterine irritability called for strict bed rest. I blamed it on my age, just short of thirty-eight I should have expected to endure some difficulty with my pregnancy. And, why wouldn't my uterus be irritable? Years of indecision and stalling to conceive, to allow my body to become a vessel for new life, that in of itself probably warranted some form of anger, resentment and maybe even some twisted form of retribution. Not from my husband, mother, sister, but from my uterus no less.

Sometimes I would pretend he wasn't growing in my belly, wholly dependent on me to carry him through to term. It was too much to bear. The contractions became constant throughout the day—a trip to the bathroom, precariously leaning over the bathroom sink to rinse my neglected teeth with a shot of mouthwash (as I could no longer put a toothbrush between my lips for fear of the gag reflex); the clipping of a rogue hangnail from my big toe, and the most significant undertaking, an attempt to run a razor along my legs to ward off the inch of black hairs growing with a vengeance—another boon of pregnancy—bountiful hair growth. And then, one of the above and/or any combination thereof, led to a series of premature visits to labor and delivery.

At the onset of each series of uterine irritations, the second-guessing, bargaining and circular conversations void of logic would commence. Should we go to the hospital? Or keep counting the waves of contractions; noting the strength, length and frequency as the pressure cramped my stomach. When my doctor instructed me to start counting my contractions, it seemed to be a fairly simple task, but weeks later it turned into an all consuming ritual. I had filled two full notebooks in the last week. And how to discern Braxton

Hicks from real, true, honest-to-goodness the baby is coming out right now, call 911, scream for your husband contractions—the doctor said true labor contractions would come every 3-5 minutes, lasting 60 to 90 seconds each, for at least one hour and getting stronger. Well, I had already had that scenario beat. Multiple times. Each premature visit to labor and delivery, following the examinations, cervix checks and fetal monitoring the nurses determined it was false labor. However grateful my husband and I were with the knowledge that the baby was still safe and growing, I couldn't help but feel somewhat ashamed. Ashamed for the mad dash to the hospital, hanging my head as my husband escorted me though the labor and delivery corridor past the nurses' station and outside the automatic doors.

The interrogation by my husband didn't help matters. *Drink more water. How much had I drunk today?* he asked. The water—always the fucking water. I swallowed it by the gallons. Was he suggesting that I was at fault for the contractions? Jesus, if I could stop them I would. Take another deep breath, calm down. The medicated regimen had begun one week earlier with Nifedipine, actually indicated for high blood pressure and heart disease, but used for I.U. for its ability to smooth muscle cells. It smoothed nothing for me. The follow-up drug was Indomethacin, which slowed the contractions, but limited to 48 hours, so this was merely a short-term fix for my uterus, like bribing a petulant child with the promise of a toy if they would just behave while mom completed her trip to the supermarket. Now I was popping 2.5 mg of Terbutaline every four hours around the clock, the most recent prescribed antidote.

Ironically, pregnancy was supposed to be the time to double-up on sleep before the all-night feedings and diaper changes commenced. Even the term 'bed rest' was a misnomer in my particular case, for minutes after ingesting the little off-white pills I experienced similar symptoms as a meth-freak would after snorting a line of yellowed powder: jitteriness, accelerated heart-rate and teeth-grinding. It was awful. But it curbed the contractions. All I could hope for was a manageable civility between me and my volatile uterus. My husband paced back and forth. Perplexed, he grabbed my notebook from the dresser at the side of our bed amidst the medications, half-eaten granola bars, thermos of ice water, saltines and T.V. remote. Then fear begat anger and I watched his brow furrow at his powerlessness over my irritable uterus.

So we went to the hospital. As usual, I was all apologies. Again, feeling like a fraud, the boy or rather the girl that cried wolf. It was my fourth visit that month. A young male intake wheeled me though the hospital hallways toward labor and delivery. He probably barely had his first drink of legal alcohol, I thought, finding myself keeping my head down, embarrassed at my neglected roots as he smiled and waved to the other orderlies. I felt simultaneously hideous, incompetent, and annoyed for succumbing to vanity even under these circumstances. As we turned the corner, the familiar closed door of the NICU appeared. Paper cut-outs of storks carrying babies bundled in blue and pink blankets danced across the windows darkened to passersby by closed blinds.

Once inside our room, I found some slight comfort, allowing my ripening belly to fall with gravity onto the bed. I exhaled slowly, hoping someone would come soon and protect my baby. The room was cold, but at least in the side position I had a reprieve from our growing boy, no more pressure on my bladder, lower back or in-between my rib cage. He probably needed the repositioning as well, I thought, imagining him swimming free-style through my amniotic fluid.

Our assigned nurse abruptly pushed open the door to our room, clipboard in hand. She ordered me to remove all of my clothes and pushed one of those open back nightgowns into my hands.

"You're drinking your water?"

I nodded.

"Staying in bed?"

I nodded.

"No sex?"

My husband nodded.

She jotted our responses onto her paperwork then took both hands and pushed me further onto my side, freeing one hand to throw an elastic belt around my stomach from underneath—some sort of lasso trick she had probably refined over the years—strapping two devices to my stomach, one to measure the fetal heartbeat, the other to measure the intensity and duration of the contractions. She turned away and moved her fingers across the monitor, aligning a new roll of paper from beneath, all the while eyeing the machine with each erratic beep. Initially I thought she was sick with a cold as she continued to snort and wiggle her nose while pacing around at my bedside, but then I realized it was merely a tic of annoyance, further displayed as she positioned her left arm behind my back and moved the thick black elastic band up a little, then down, then refastened it tighter when the whirring of the baby's heart beat *whoosha-whoosha-whoosha* finally came into agreement with her machine.

"I need you to pull up your gown and scoot your bottom to the edge of the bed, please," she ordered.

"Come on," she said, patting her hand against the end of the bed, "keep moving."

Flat on my back, with my legs spread wide open trembling from atrophy, I didn't know how much longer I could stay in position. As she pushed two, three, or maybe four of her latexed fingers toward my cervix, she addressed my husband, "You helping mom out at home, dad?" I couldn't see my husband, but I knew he was pissed.

The nurse then warned us of the hazards of dehydration, which was one of the great paradoxes of the whole I.U. treatment plan since drinking eight liters of water a day saturated one's bladder, resulting in numerous trips to the bathroom and the cumulative trips resulted in uterine contractions. I was caught between the proverbial Scylla and Charybdis.

Attempting to block out her proselytizing and not show a trace of hostility for fear she would retaliate (being in such close proximity to my unborn); I fixed my eyes onto the ceiling, focusing on the light above. Just focus on the white light. Light is good. Holy, pure white light, I thought, at least until I noticed a spray of lifeless mosquitoes littering the curve of the opaque light cover. In a blink, God's divine light transformed into dead bugs. Who knew how long they had been there. Their little bits of legs, and wings withered from the scorching fluorescent bulbs. *Whoosha-whoosha-whoosha.* And for a moment I mourned the cruel fiery death of the winged creatures.

"Cervix still long and thick," she cleared her throat, snorted and reached even further. The pressure of her hand inside caused me to flinch back to protect my core from her deliberate fingers. "No dilation and minimal effacement," she finally pronounced, promptly peeling off the gloves and tossing them into the trash bin to join all of the other used L&D paraphernalia.

I pulled myself up from the edge of the bed, grabbing my balled-up jumbo-sized pink cotton panties, relieved at the exam results. We could go home now and finish off last night's pint of Ben & Jerry's Chunky Monkey basking in this short reprieve. Our little guy was still intact, at least for the time being. Before I could pull my underwear up over my belly, the nurse put her hand up as if to cease any further motion.

"Have you ever heard of brain bleeds?" she posed, as she examined the printout from the monitor. "Happened to a twenty-six week old that we had in here just last week. Mother was a smoker . . . but it has occurred on my watch many a time in my twenty-five years."

My stomach dropped as she continued with her cautionary tale. "Babies really need that extra time to develop . . . remember that. We don't want to see you in here again," she ordered. "You don't want your boy riding the short bus—do you? I see you've at least had the doses of glutocorticoids. I've seen those NICU babies on breathing tubes for months and it's not pretty."

And it was conclusive. She was a sadist. A sadist hidden behind the pretext of offering sound medical counsel. Brain bleeds. Short bus. I swallowed back a burp of bitter bile as cries of new life echoed from across the hall.

As I lay on the gurney watching the gel ooze across my belly, I told myself I couldn't name him mine. Not yet. Not at thirty weeks. But he emerged onto the tiny screen in all of his black and white grainy glory—the silhouette of his bulbous head and nip of a nose reminiscent of Schultz's endearing cartoon character Charlie Brown. I imagined a thin spray of curlicues sprouting from the top of his head, waving his little hand at us, hoping the football would not get pulled out from under him. And then the radiologist pointed out the four chambers of his tiny heart. Strong and steady. *Whoosha-whoosha-whoosha.*

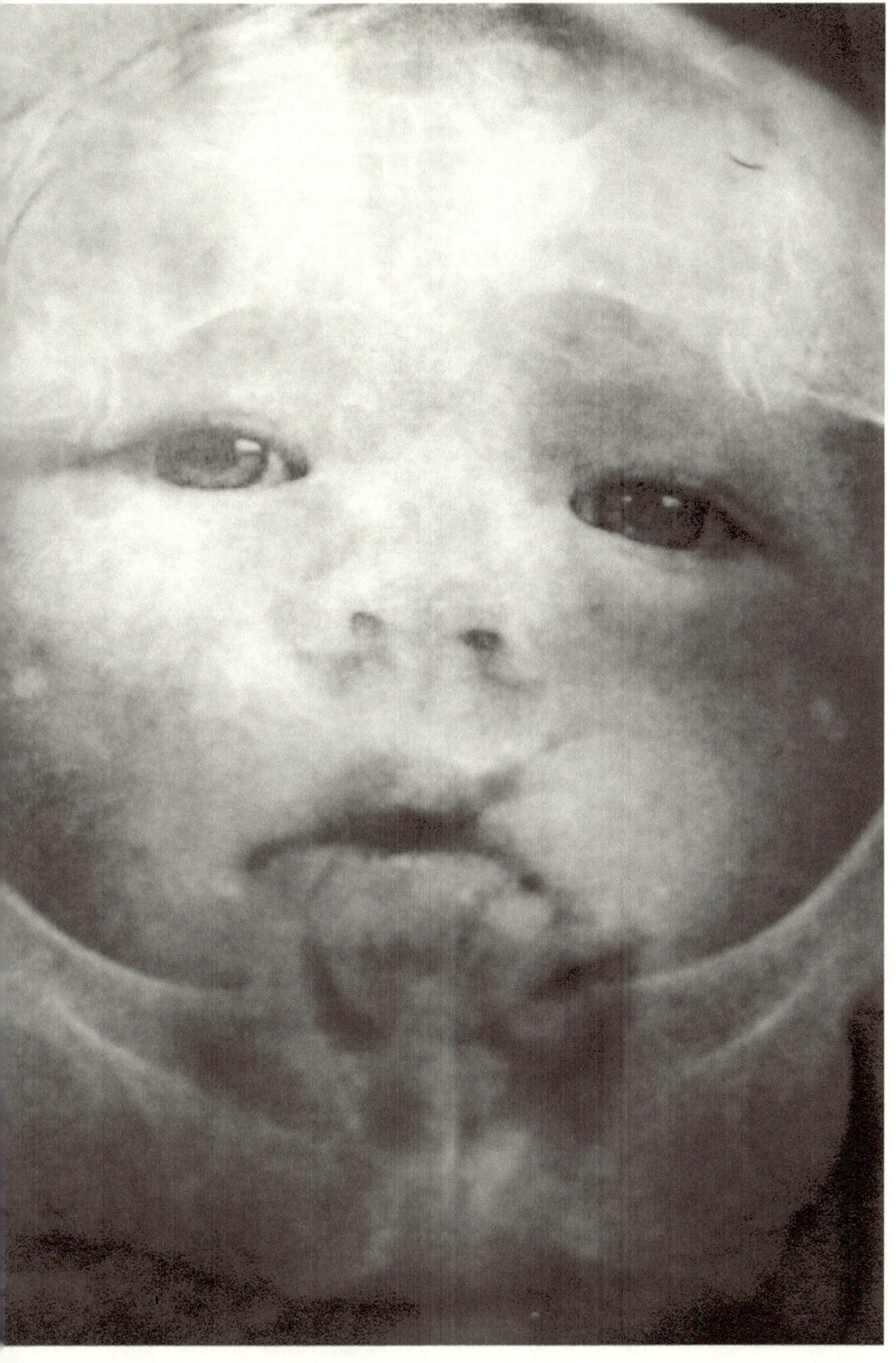

JOAN PHILLIPS

THE HOME FOR UNWED MOTHERS

I was sixteen
They let us put one wish for our child
Into the folder
Of course there was no guarantee
The adoptive family could or would honor it
I said I just wanted him in a Christian home

I was sixteen
I made the choice to give him up
They knocked me out for the delivery
I didn't see him for five days
They don't want you to bond
We weren't supposed to take a picture when we saw them
But every girl left that home with a picture
Of her baby

I was sixteen
I waited sixteen more years to ever have my own children
I didn't want him to think it didn't matter to me
I wanted my life to be worth it
I just needed to know I did something

She is almost through with her doctorate
She has two beautiful little daughters
She has a letter saying her son has registered
And might want contact with her
She realizes she never gave him up
And never will
All the letter says is he lives in Texas somewhere
And his name is Christian

SARA LIPPMANN

GIRL

Here is where she waits to get one. It is a particular place—this waiting room—for particular services although there are no visible markers. No activity clogging the sidewalk, gruesome posters slung from anyone's neck. Instead there is an elevator and a hallway and a door that opens onto the predictable hum of fluorescence, a waiting room like any other. Absent only are Matchbox cars careening along the rim of the coffee table, the clumsy presence of strollers. A ground-in trail of snack puffs.

The twins she has left at home.

The wallpaper is floral pastel, like what one might expect in a suburban family's powder room. Once she locked herself in Stephanie Quinn's downstairs powder room. She was sixteen and high on mushrooms but sitting here now she remembers how the petals wove and sparkled that night, how she lay there on the floor, holding on to it all for a while before twisting the knob to show Stephanie Quinn: how beautiful.

There was no sex at sixteen and while there were other things, she was considered a good girl for this reason. The room is filled with girls, slouched in chairs, their heads resting on the shoulders of mothers, aunts, older sisters. Girls sucking the strings of their hooded sweatshirts, sucking until the wet cotton squeaks in their mouths, hoods pulled tight, compressing their skulls. They are not like her and yet she is one of them.

"Hang on Sloopy" comes on the oldies station and two girls in full wigs spin heels straight from the club.

It is eleven o'clock in the morning. Her husband has taken off work. He is reading the newspaper on his handheld device. The radio plays. Heat spreads from her ears, stamping down her throat, like how she used to get while giving an oral presentation when no one was paying attention. She squeezes her husband's arm but he has a call and stands up to take it outside. Lowering her eyes, she scans the waists in the waiting room: a tight peach t-shirt, a midriff baring a belly ring, a cheap blazer stretched over a bulge.

There are fathers here, too.

A vase rests on the windowsill full of cloudy water. Lilies. Their scent could nauseate her even when fresh, but these flowers have started to turn, stamens spilling rust along the ledge. Bile rises but then her name is called and she reports for the transaction, her credit card swiped through a machine. There are receipts and consent forms and handouts, poorly copied, detailing risks and side effects, a slip with prescriptions to fill.

She signs off on everything.

The office assistant asks if there is anything else.

She shakes her head. The doctor had ordered a twelve-hour fast and now she feels like she does on Yom Kippur. Her nose tingles. She fights it as she's been fighting for weeks but she is failing. A nurse with a cross pendant appears at her side.

"Something wrong, sugar?"

"It's only," she says, halting. "I am a mother."

The nurse tells her try not to think of it like that.

Her voice breaks, "you don't understand," but before she can whisper "already" there is her husband, kissing her forehead and saying, "What did I miss?" She looks at him through smeary eyes and he says, "Remember, this is your decision." Just like that he's excused himself as if to clarify: this is her problem. She could stop it but where would that leave them? The nurse with the crucifix balls up a wad of tissues and offers them up as a bouquet. Her husband invites her to blow.

"Isn't that sweet," the nurse speaks in a tone used on small children. Rubs her back and it is embarrassing. "You two are a breath of fresh air."

A door opens and her husband turns. The nurse throws out her hand like a crossing guard. "The girls in there are half-naked." His protest is thin but at least there is a protest and at least he is here, she reminds herself, as her husband retreats to the waiting room and she follows the nurse down the corridor labeled "no men allowed."

The changing area feels like the dressing room of a discount women's department store. Vainly she'd fretted over what to wear this morning, not wanting to look too prim or too casual. Too much like a mommy. The twins had clomped around the closet in her shoes, draping rejected pieces around them like boas. Squealing; "look at me." Once the disposable gown is tied, she gathers her belongings into a pile. It is freezing. There are paper bags on her feet. One girl—no, a woman—looks at her nipples begging through and indicates a row of lockers, their keys attached to springy neon rings.

"Girl," the woman says. "Just wait for that tea." The air conditioner grunts and she shivers, shuffling to her locker, sliding the key chain over her wrist.

A new waiting room. More girls. Fidgeting in their chairs, thumbing outdated issues of *Prevention* and *Country Home*. One speaks into a smuggled cell phone, loudly, so it is impossible to mishear the words "dilation" and "sticks." Another picks a scab on her arm. It's taking forever and the light screams down at her. The gown provides insufficient coverage. Tugging at it, she has begun to feel dizzy so when a girl asks, "what time is it?" she almost says, "naptime."

Inside she does as she's told: dangles her ass off the table, presses her feet into stirrups. The doctor enters. His nose and mouth are masked but she recognizes his eyes from his website. This man could sell her a bridge. He stands at her feet, waving a wand, and says with an accent: "First we need to confirm what is there."

She is grateful for the nurse anesthetist. It will not take much. Only yesterday the twins had crashed toy carriages, dolls expunged in a lifeless heap, and begged her for a real baby brother. They are not quite three, her girls, but she's settled on a tea set and pair of wings for them each as consolation. The anesthetist rolls out his questions of consciousness. Her teeth clatter.

"Relax," the anesthetist says.

The gas hisses and she breathes; "that a girl," she hears as the cup closes down on her face.

Again with the flowers, faded border. Drop ceiling. A room lined like a convent with beds; still, more are needed. The nurse rushes to move her. To accommodate the ones who must wait. The girl beside her is sobbing; the girl across rises and spills. Now that it is over she is ravenous—sucked and pink and scraped clean—and the only thing she can think is what to eat.

The girls spoke of abortion tea for good reason. Blend of Lipton, chamomile flower, peppermint; whatever bags are left over. Brewed in a samovar and served thick with honey in a Styrofoam cup. The nurse brings it to her chair in recovery, along with two pills to help out the cramping. Her crucifix winks and here comes a pad used for housebreaking puppies. The nurse coos: "slide this under your bum." She is so hungry the hot tea is heaven going down, fills her right up, as if it were all she could want.

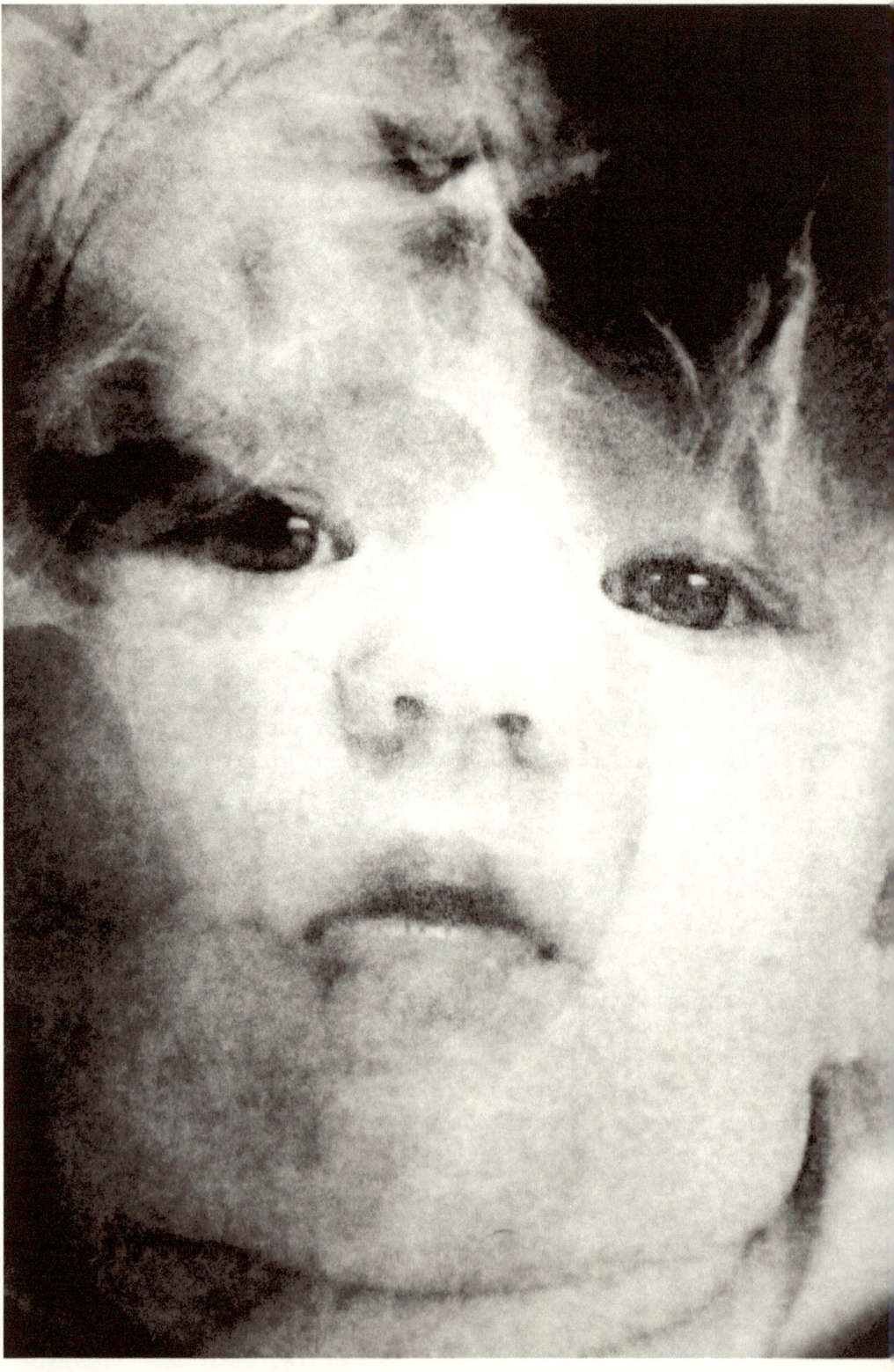

MICHELE MARKARIAN

DON'T YOU WANT THIS BABY?

Garine sat in the waiting room of the doctor's office, thinking, is this really happening?

That morning, as she was getting ready for art class, it occurred to her that although her period was only three days late, her breasts were leaden and swollen with a familiar heavy ache. Garine was loathe to take a pregnancy test—at forty-five, she had suffered a miscarriage last year, and was so desperate for another baby that she dared not even hope for it. Yet there would be company for dinner, and most likely one or two bottles of wine . . .

Garine noted the time. She took the test stick out of the box and after peeing on it, laid it gently on the vanity. She washed her hands, made her bed, looked at the clock. Five minutes had passed. Garine checked on the stick. She was pregnant.

Her husband was at work and her six-year-old son was dressing for camp. She wanted to tell him that he was going to be a big brother, but thought better of it. Yet one pregnancy book she'd read recently said that it was important to tell people right way, so that the child will know it's welcome.

She dropped her son off at camp and called her husband on his cellphone. "Guess what?" she said, and when he couldn't guess, she told him.

"Really?" The disbelief in his voice was audible. It was pretty incredible, considering her age. "Did you feel this or something?"

"No, but I know we have people coming tonight, and I didn't want to drink if there were a chance," she said.

"Are you sure? Did you call the doctor? Maybe you should get another test?"

"I'm definitely pregnant," said Garine. "I'll set up an appointment with the doctor and call you later, okay?"

"Good luck. I love you," said her husband, before hanging up.

Feeling like it might be real, she called her best friend, Julie. Julie had had her only child at the age of forty-four. "Guess what?" she said, trying to sound light.

"You're pregnant," said Julie.

Maybe Julie knowing this immediately was a good sign, a sign that the baby's spirit was strong, thought Garine. "I probably shouldn't have said anything. It's so early. I mean, what if I lose this one, too?"

"You won't," said Julie firmly, and Garine almost felt reassured.

Garine walked to art class, and tried to feel settled and at peace with the pregnancy, but didn't. Maybe it had something to do with last year's miscarriage. Maybe it had something to do with the fact that her husband, cautious by nature, didn't seem to be doing handsprings through the telephone, the way she hoped he would. At any rate, when she got back from art class and went to pee, she noticed a bright red spot the size of a quarter on her underpants and called the doctor. That's when they advised her to come in immediately.

"Garine Hagopian?" A small, trim nurse with pale skin and a black perm spiked with gray stood in the doorway. "You can come with me."

The nurse led Garine into a smaller office in the back. She showed her the bathroom where to urinate, then took Garine's blood pressure. Garine noticed that the last name on the nurse's nametag was Armenian, just like hers. "Are you Armenian?" she asked, just to make conversation and hide her nervousness. The nurse didn't seem Armenian. She was too prim, too tidy. The Armenian women Garine grew up with were unwittingly spilling over with emotion and intensity.

"Um hmm," said the nurse as she swabbed Garine's arm before taking blood. She was one of those people who carried an air of self-contained tranquility about them—her movements, the way she spoke, all seemed to float on cotton swabs.

"I'm afraid something's wrong," blurted Garine. The bloodstain didn't feel right. There were no cramps, her breasts felt bulbous and full, but there was that damn bloodstain.

"Oh no. This is perfectly normal," said the nurse in her calm, Buddha-like way. "Breathe in." She gently inserted a syringe.

Garine looked away. She hated watching the clear syringe change to dark red. "Is it?" asked Garine in disbelief. It didn't feel normal.

"Lots of people have bleeding." Her words were tighter now, more compressed. The nurse withdrew the syringe that was in Garine's arm. She pressed tightly with a cotton pad on the spot where she withdrew the blood. "This kind of thing happens all the time. It's perfectly normal."

Panic rose in Garine. The nurse's insistence that vaginal bleeding during pregnancy was perfectly normal was almost surreal. She was willing to believe her, but needed more proof. "Really? It doesn't feel normal."

The nurse removed the cotton gauze and put a bandaid over the prick. "Why? Don't you want this baby?"

Garine looked at the nurse, her bad perm, her serenely closed off face with the prim mouth and wondered if she'd heard right.

"Don't you want this baby?" Garine sat, stunned. Was there hostility behind the loving gestures—the cotton swab, the bandaid, the gentle pressing down? Garine couldn't be sure.

Later on that week, when it was confirmed that Garine had indeed lost the baby before it had even begun, Garine thought about the nurse. "Don't you want this baby?" She thought about the nurse when the doctor wouldn't schedule a D & E until she was sure the fetus wouldn't eliminate itself, which of course it didn't—Garine knew that her body wouldn't let a fetus go so easily, even though it was dead. "Don't you want this baby?" And years later, when it was too late to have a baby, and Garine knew that wanting a baby had nothing to do with getting one, and that sometimes life just doesn't give you what you want, she thought of that nurse's impertinence and she realized that despite her better judgment, the nurse had cut her deeply, had given her doubt.

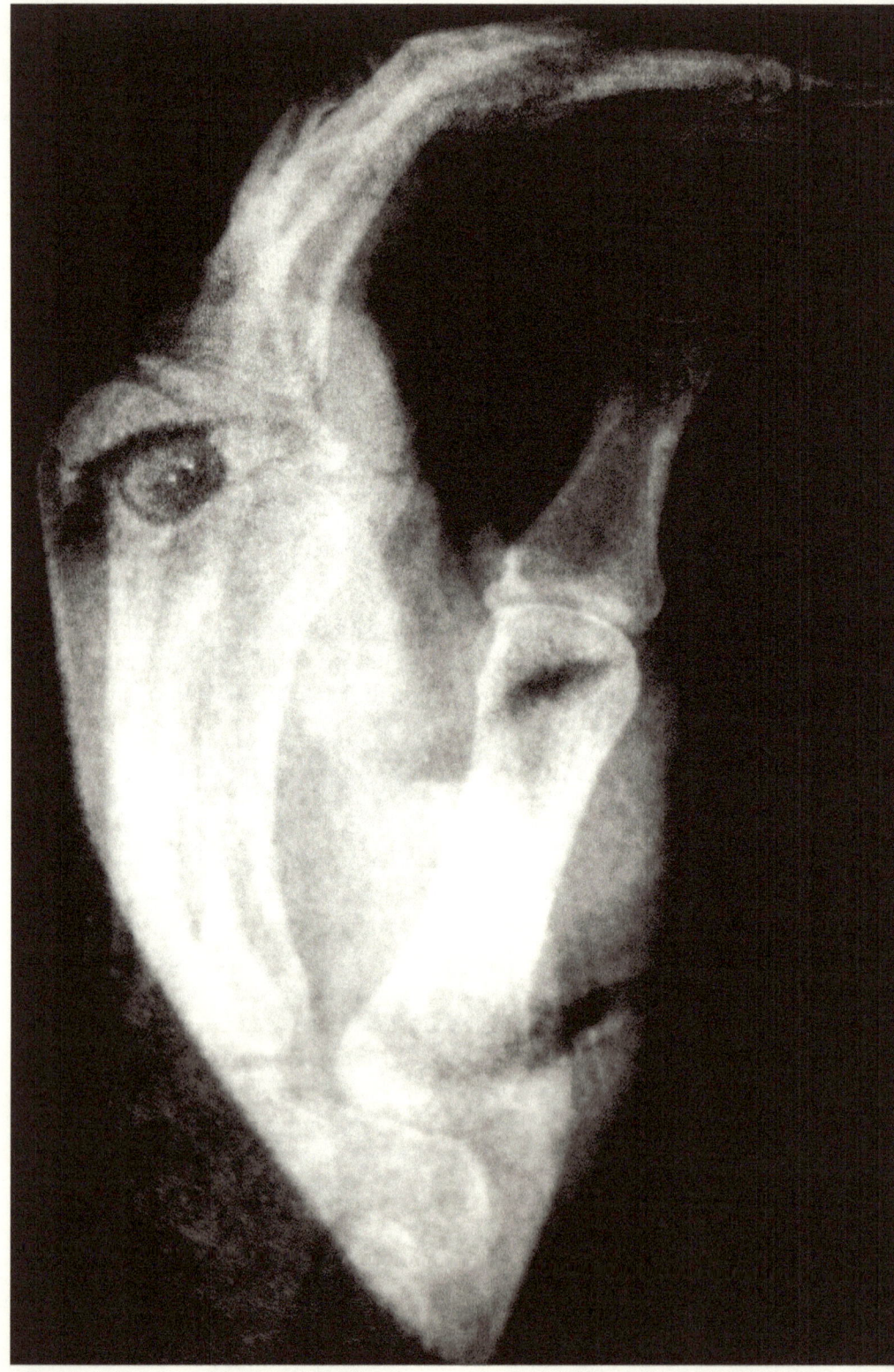

V
ERRORS

JANE HERSCHLAG

THE METAPHOR OF ILLNESS

Submission beaten into her young body,
self-defense ringed out of her neck,
by age three she lost
all tools to oppose.
                    * * *
Mt. Sinai's Chief Dental Surgeon
supervises, as his student hacks
at her impacted wisdom tooth.
Dr. X returns to see the progress—
he removes the wrongly inserted
intravenous needle and corrects it.
Occasionally he checks on her.
Ninety minutes later he decides,
to complete the extraction.

A month of days crawls by, still only able
to open her mouth enough
to slip baby food past her teeth,
Dr. X says, It's just psychic.
Chew bubble gum.
Two more months and two other dentists
yield no healing or diagnosis.

Exhausted, she sinks deeper into her pain
and tear-soaked pillow—
assessing herself mentally ill;
zombie-like she cooks and cares
for two pre-schoolers.

Fall tinges summer,
now throat pain rivals jaw pain,
her voice peeps like a chick's.

She drags one heavy leg in front
of the other, to the internist's office.
A blood test— instant admission
into Columbia Presbyterian Hospital.
An X-ray technician pries her swollen jaw apart,
places film on the wound. The head and neck surgeon says,
You have a 50 percent chance of surviving
this jaw bone infection that has spread.
If you make it through the next twenty-four hours
you'll soon walk out of here. I won't get involved,
but you should sue the dental surgeon.
Don't ask me to testify.
　　　　* * *

Two decades later she discovers,
her body knew what her mind forgot—
that dental student's assault
echoed her father's oral rapes
as her mother, like Dr. X, absented herself.
More than tears, that surgery incited
a flood of white blood cells
that nested in her bone marrow.
　　　　* * *

Her history excised from repression
by her therapist,
the open pages of her journal,
stanzas of her poetry—
after cancer, diabetes,
and Sjorgren syndrome
her white blood count
is no longer elevated,
her immune system
almost tests normal.

GROWING UP IN A WAR-ZONE-HOME

yields odd benefits.
Learned vigilance protects.

When Doctor Segal says,
There are insufficient cells
but the test results are benign,
come back in six months,

I know, my judgment was right,
lauded as tops, he's senile—
three needles thrust in
don't yield enough cells.

Not lured into complacency
by the bait of benign,
I don't wait six months
for my enemy to grow,
I demand another referral.

Both thyroid lobes riddled with cancer—
my metabolic General is excised
before rampant cells travel.
Parathyroid glands and lymph nodes clean—
no need for radioactive iodine.

FREDRICKA R. MAISTER

DIAGNOSING THE DOCTOR: FEAR OF TRUTH

A physician admitting culpability and expressing regret for a medical mistake?

My medical ordeal began when I awoke one morning to a barrage of black web-like strands floating in my field of vision. Aware that 'floaters' could be symptomatic of a detached retina, I immediately contacted my trusted ophthalmologist who 'squeezed' me in during the one hour he would be in his office following up on surgical patients.

To enable him to perform a thorough examination, he dilated my eyes a number of times. The examination proceeded without a hitch and my retina proved to be intact. I would just have to make friends with my floaters until they disappeared.

My vision was blurry afterwards, which the medical staff said was to be expected, but once outside in the sunlight I found myself walking in a foggy landscape inhabited by ghostly figures. I could not see street signs or distinguish between red and green lights. I had to ask people where I was in my own neighborhood! Terrified that a car would hit me, I chased 'human shapes' as they crossed busy intersections.

By the time I arrived home my eyes were stinging. Anxious that something had gone awry, I asked my concierge to dial the doctor's office for me, as I could not see the numbers on the telephone. The doctor's receptionist assured me that my experience was normal and that cold compresses would ease the burning sensation.

Despite the compresses, my eyelids were swelling up. My eyes would not stay open. And I was in agony! I thought I might have been allergic to the eye drops or anesthetic used during the examination. I called the doctor's office again. The physician's assistant doubted that I was having an allergic reaction and told me to use warm compresses.

As the hours passed, the pain intensified. I called the doctor's office a third time, insisting, "Something is wrong!" The physician's assistant barked accusingly, "Well, I don't know what happened between the time you left the office and got home!" He told me to continue using warm compresses.

In exasperation, I phoned the doctor at his other office. The doctor, via his secretary, told me to apply cold compresses to alleviate my discomfort, which he attributed to his rigorous eye examination, and to see him the next day if the problem persisted.

With eyes reduced to slits and eyelids inflamed and bulging, I showed up the next morning without an appointment. No one seemed surprised to see me.

"Abrasions. Just what I thought," the doctor said on immediate examination. The cornea in both eyes had been scratched! The doctor mumbled something about the anesthetic on my eyelids forming icicles in the frigid weather that might have rubbed against the cornea.

On hearing the diagnosis, I fluctuated between anxiety about losing my eyesight and anger at the ophthalmologist and his staff for: allowing me to go out, heavily dilated with fresh anesthetic, into the winter air; ignoring the seriousness of my condition which I reported in four phone calls, and failing to disclose that a possible medical error had occurred for which they were sorry.

Without a satisfactory explanation, I obsessed over what could have caused the corneal abrasions in both my eyes. My childhood ophthalmologist, in consultation with my physician uncle, suggested that the problem might have occurred due to a sudden jerky motion by the doctor (he might have been rushed because of his tight schedule) or by me (it's not easy to still the eyes during a prolonged exam). A friend knew someone whose cornea became scratched when eye drops were improperly administered (I certainly had my share of drops that day). Or maybe, after all, frozen anesthetic was the culprit (my eyelids did feel increasingly heavy as I walked home).

When I asked my ophthalmologist point-blank, "What do you think caused this?" he evasively replied, "I could guess, but let's just get you better."

The doctor's withholding of information and disregard for my right to know what he knew or suspected smacked of 'cover up' and only exacerbated my emotional distress. Feelings of anger and betrayal, coupled with my frustration at the slow healing process (one eye resolved overnight, but 'the crater' in the other eye would take weeks), later spilled out in the waiting room when I told a longtime patient whose eyesight the doctor had saved what had happened to me. My behavior may have been inappropriate, but I needed to vent.

All that said, I still think my ophthalmologist was probably an excellent and competent physician. He was also a fallible human being who did not intend to put me in harm's way. Most importantly, thanks to his and his staff's diligent care, my eyes healed, my vision fully restored.

However, despite my physical recovery, I had unresolved emotional issues that undermined our patient-physician relationship. How could I continue to trust a physician who would not disclose a possible medical error truthfully and compassionately?

Out of fear of litigation or embarrassment, my ophthalmologist would not even apologize. If only he had said, "I'm sorry," I could have forgiven him. Case closed.

ANNE WEBSTER

THE NURSE I CAN'T FORGET

"Larry, I'm so afraid." I sat on the side of a hospital bed, leaning against my husband, as he stood beside me.

"I don't know what to do," Larry said. In the mirror over the sink I could see the reflection of his face. It held an emotion I'd never seen in our forty years together—fear.

Tears slid down my cheeks as I looked at the wall calendar. It was September 26, three months before my sixtieth birthday, one I might never see. When I had gotten up to the bathroom, my swollen legs had splayed like bowling pins, and the buttons on my pajama top threatened to pop. I gasped for each breath while my heart ricocheted around in my chest.

"See if you can find a nurse. I hit the call light ten minutes ago, but they don't bother to answer."

"I'll get someone. They won't ignore me again."

"What do you need?" asked the sour-faced nurse who followed Larry into the room a few minutes later.

"I want to be weighed."

"Lie still. These beds have built-in scales." She fiddled with the controls. "Hmm, 153, does that sound about right?"

"It's twenty-eight pounds over my admitting weight four days ago." I fought to keep the shrillness out of my voice. "Look at my legs. I have four plus pitting edema." I pressed an ankle, leaving a deep imprint. "I can hardly breathe, and my heartbeat is irregular, but no one has listened to my chest, I've been here five days, and I'm getting worse every hour."

How could I, an experienced nurse, have become a victim of such sloppy nursing? I had attended nursing school and later worked at this very hospital. Since a diagnosis of Crohn's disease forced me to give up my job on the coronary step-down unit, I had only visited the hospital as an outpatient, but I'd never lost my pride in having been on staff here and in the excellent standard of care the hospital offered.

That loyalty had left me both dismayed and hurt when I'd been admitted the week before with severe anemia due to an incorrectly prescribed immunosuppressant drug. The nurses on the med-surg unit where I was sent from the Emergency Department had failed to follow basic protocols, like performing frequent vital signs during blood administration or delivering medications on time. They didn't bother to supply my room with the paper towels necessary for the reverse isolation which had been ordered, nor did they do routine assessments, exams which would have red-flagged my increasing breathing problems, edema, and arrhythmic heart. I was sure that my hours were numbered. I'd seen it happen to patients all too often not to recognize the signs.

I heard a tap on the door, and my daughter-in-law walked in. Julie, a nurse practitioner who worked in another part of the hospital, stared at me for a moment, and ran from the room. I would later learn that she had rushed to the Nursing Administration office and burst into tears. The President of Nursing had contacted my doctor, and the nurse-administrator for the Medical-Surgical division personally delivered my morning medications.

Soon a lung specialist arrived. He frowned as he listened to my chest. "I'm ordering a chest X-ray, but I know what it will show—pneumonia. We're moving you to ICU."

Because of Julie's intervention, I had a chance at living.

I slid from the stretcher onto the waiting ICU bed. The maneuver left me panting worse than I had earlier, even with five liters of oxygen going. I sat up straight and hit the button to raise the head of the bed. To lie flat would be to smother.

"Hi, I'm Laura," said a pretty brunette. "Remember me?"

"Sure. I worked with you a couple of times when you were pulled to the step-down unit. It's nice to see a familiar face."

"How are you feeling?" she asked as she stuck monitor leads to my chest and placed a glowing clamp on an index finger to measure my oxygen saturation levels.

"Pretty rough, I can't get enough air."

"It's the pneumonia. We'll give you a diuretic to get rid of some of the excess fluid. That should help your breathing." She glanced up at the erratic pattern threading across the cardiac monitor. "How long have you been having this arrhythmia?"

"Who knows? They didn't have monitors on the other unit. I told them about my irregular pulse, but nobody did anything."

"Dr. Myers, a cardiologist, is coming to do a consult on you. He'll get this sorted out."

"Good. He's the best. I used to work with him."

"Give me a few minutes to go over your chart. In the meanwhile, call me if you need anything."

"I'm going to ask your doctor to order some renal-dose dobutamine," Laura said when she returned.

"But that drug is used in kidney failure. I thought my kidneys were okay." I took as deep a breath as my soupy lungs would allow. "What's my BUN-Creatinine ratio?" An elevation in that blood test would indicate acute renal failure.

"It's thirty-two, twice as high as normal." While Laura talked, her hands never stopped moving—smoothing the sheets, checking the IV connections, adjusting my oxygen.

"One more thing," Laura's forehead wrinkled with concern. "You must be very careful and let us assist you when you get up to the bathroom. With your low platelet count, you would bleed to death if you so much as stubbed your toe. Remember, we are here to help you."

As the door closed behind her, I relaxed for the first time since I'd been admitted. At last, a nurse who cared, one who might be able to stem the tide of negative events that had brought me to this unit.

"You look tired," Laura said the next morning.

"It's hard to sleep sitting straight up, but I can't breathe if I lower the bed."

"No wonder you can't rest." Laura frowned over her stethoscope as she leaned me forward to listen to my lungs. "These wrinkles in the sheets are cutting into your back."

"Do you think you could get up a few minutes so I can fix your bed?" She helped me to the chair, deftly keeping my two IV lines and four cardiac leads from tangling, quickly stripped the bed, and smoothed on fresh sheets.

Fresh sheets. No one had volunteered to change my bed once on the other unit, and now I had my second set in twelve hours. I continued to marvel as Laura brought a pan of warm water and washed my hands and face, rubbed lotion on my back, which, after lying for so long in one position to breathe, had felt permanently imprinted with wrinkles. When she settled me into bed, I sank back gratefully.

"How is that? Is there anything else I can do?" she asked.

"Thank you, no. This clean bed feels great."

As Laura tiptoed out of the room, I looked at her with new eyes. I had worked with her, but one nurse never knows what kind of job another nurse does, because nurses rarely go into a patient's room if they aren't assigned to that patient. I'd had no idea that Laura gave such excellent care.

The week I was in Intensive Care, Laura proved to be the norm. Joy, a Philippine nurse, made me crazy at first by bowing and saying, "Yes, ma'am, Miss Anne," each time she came into my room. But her expert attention rivaled Laura's care, as did Ellen's, another nurse with whom I'd worked. Ruth, who shared my mother's name, comforted me in the same way my mother often had, by cupping my hand in hers as she talked to me.

After a week in ICU the pneumonia lessened and my blood counts began to rise. I was transferred to a regular bed in a hematology unit, and the isolation lifted. For the first time I felt hopeful that I might live to see my grandchildren grow up.

Although I would never understand the lax treatment I'd received by the nurses on Five East, those bad experiences had been offset by nurses like Laura, the intelligent interventions and selfless comfort measures provided by her and the other critical care staff. These nurses, who helped me survive a potentially deadly illness, had become my heroes. Though I wrote notes thanking each of them, I knew there would never be words enough to express my gratitude.

After nearly thirty years of taking care of patients, I had thought I'd known everything about nursing, but it was only when I became a critically ill patient that I finally understood the vital importance nurses play in recovery. Laura and her ICU colleagues made me proud to call myself "Nurse."

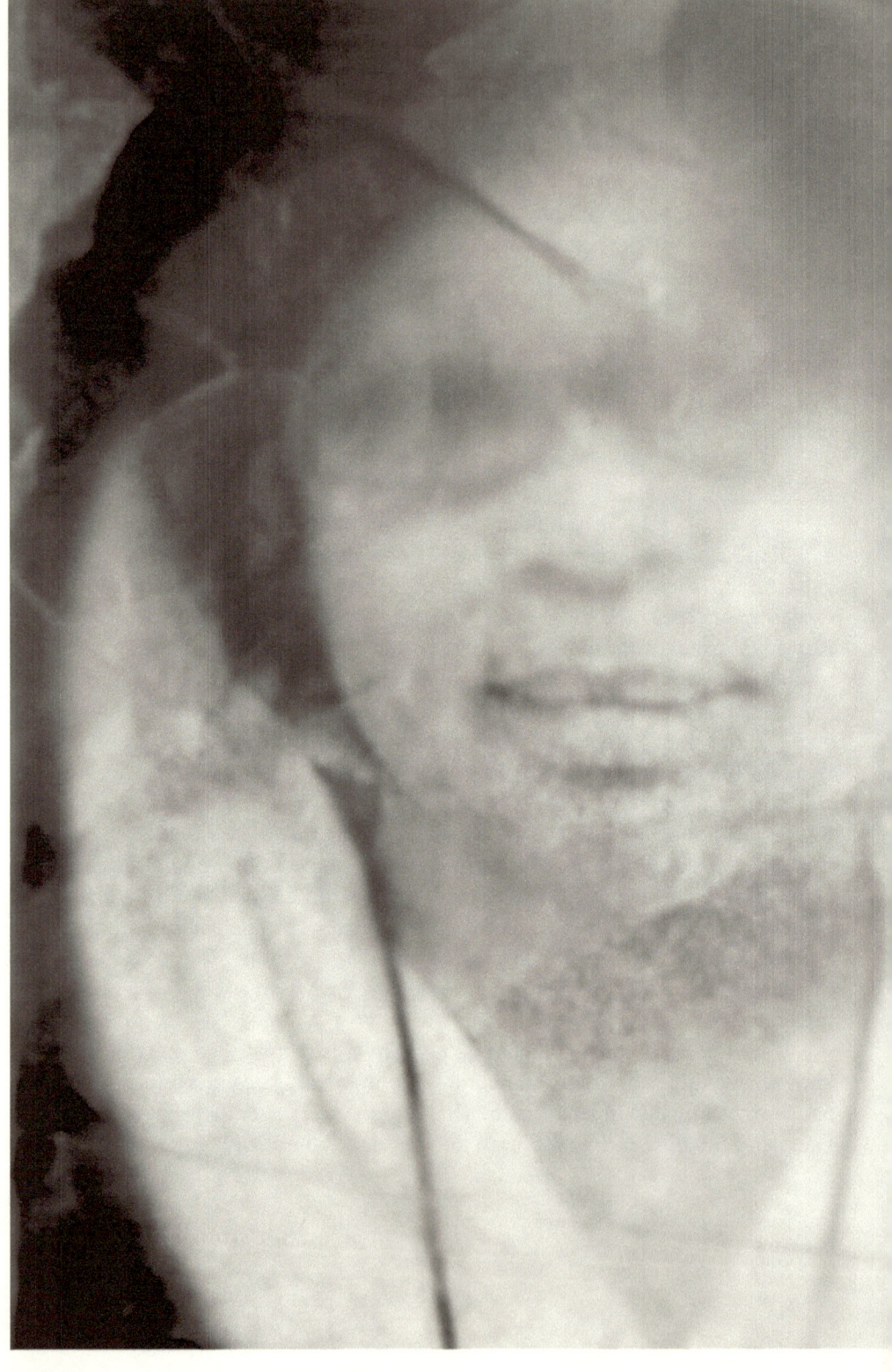

DIANE PAYNE

THESE THINGS HAPPEN

In a heavily sedated state of endless morphine, I wake up confused in a hospital bed, unsure where I am and why my leg is sliced in half and propped up on a pile of pillows. It was supposed to be an arthroscopic surgery, but something went wrong, very wrong. I ended up with major reconstructive surgery, leg split in half, staples from top to bottom.

No sooner than I begin wallowing in self-pity, my roommate, an elderly woman with a boisterous voice, starts calling me Delores, though I assure her that is not my name. "You've always been a bad girl. Lies, lies, lies. That's all you speak. You told me you were going to let me stay at home!" She throws her plastic water bottle at me. My leg is so large there's no way she could possibly miss. The pain is excruciating. I scream. She laughs.

I've only been back in this world a few hellish moments and I want to return to the world of heavy sedation. My transition from the peaceful oblivion under anesthesia to this old woman is too abrupt. I'm not even sure if all this is simply a bad dream.

A nurse hears my piercing scream down the hallway and scolds me. "Why are you screaming? Use the call button. What is this water doing all over you?"

"Delores has always been a bad girl," my roommate insists, as I lie there in a puddle of ice water, lifting the ice cubes off my blanket.

"What happened to me? I thought there would only be three holes."

The nurse frowns before answering. "You'll have to ask the doctor. There wasn't anyone waiting for you after the surgery. Why did you come alone? Now you'll have to wait until he makes his rounds tomorrow."

"May I read my chart?"

"You may, but you won't understand it."

"She never understood anything," my roommate adds. "But she

always thinks she does."

"You two are hitting it off well," the nurse laughs.

She doesn't believe me that the old woman threw her bottle at me. "Quit blaming everything on Mrs. Booth. You should be ashamed of yourself."

"Nothing but lies since the day she started to talk."

"Is this your mother?" she laughs.

The nurse turns the morphine up and finally notices that it was *her* water bottle. "Don't you hurt this girl. She just had surgery." Then out she goes, leaving me with an IV slowly dripping morphine and a roommate who keeps berating me, certain I am Delores.

Morphine does nothing to alleviate serious pain, but it does lead me into a blessed sleep. I forget about my roommate and am left alone with my drug-induced rest until a water glass comes flying across the room. There is no way the old lady can ever miss. My bed is all leg propped up on pillows. "Stop hurting me!" I scream.

"Oh, aren't you a baby, Delores? I should have hit you long ago. Then you wouldn't have turned out like this."

I try to be compassionate toward this woman, believing she is confusing me with some horrible daughter; yet, I'm not so sure she's not just a mean old lady who is angry at the world, or at least me. No one is sitting by her bedside, though I, too, am all alone in a strange city 130 miles from my home, and I'm unwilling to call the few people I know who live in Tucson because it seems like I am desperate, hoping for a visit, sympathy, which I am seeking; yet, I'd rather wait until I see the doctor. Maybe he'll release me tomorrow and everything will be fine. I thought this would be a simple outpatient surgery. I knew I might have to call someone for a ride afterwards, but I figured I'd tough it out and drive myself. Little did I know.

A new shift of nurses arrives. A young man attends to the old woman and she yells, "Rape!" He looks at me hurt, and tells her to settle down. Another nurse takes over, but not before remarking, "This is what happens when we let men become nurses." In a putrid, coddling voice, she says, "I'm here now, Mrs. Booth. Everything is okay."

"Oh, you're such a sweet girl. That man raped me."

Shaken, he comes to my bedside and I know I have an ally. "Please close the curtain between us," I plea. "She keeps throwing things at me."

"We have to get her out of here," he whispers.

But Mrs. Booth hears us. "You rotten kids. You'll go to hell," she screams while tossing the Kleenex box at me. This is the first soft thing she throws, and it bounces off the curtain.

"Mrs. Booth, you must stop throwing things or we won't be able to leave anything on your tray," he says with great patience.

"You would leave an old dying woman without water! I'm going home. My son's coming for me tonight."

During the middle of the night, another man comes to my bed and shakes me awake. He looks like a custodian and tells me I must get out of the bed and use the restroom.

I pull my blankets off and point at my leg that is too swollen to even be in a cast. "I'm not supposed to leave this bed," I say. I feel like I'm in a David Lynch movie. It's painfully surreal.

"Doctor's orders. He wants you off the bedpan and on the toilet."

"I don't even have crutches."

"You don't need them. I'll help you."

"I don't have to go to the bathroom."

"Your chart says you haven't had a bowel movement."

"I never poop in the middle of the night. I'm not leaving this bed."

"I'm taking your bedpan with me. You must get out of this bed if you want to get out of the hospital."

He storms out with my bedpan and I fall back asleep.

Later, he returns, tugging at my shoulders. "Up now. You have to walk."

The hallway is dark. I can hear a few nurses making small talk. He grabs me by the shoulders and yanks me upright. I howl. There's not enough morphine to ease the pain. My roommate turns her light on and laughs. The chatting nurses run in. "Let her be, you asshole! What are you doing? Call the supervisor, quick." The man runs off and the nurse apologizes. "You must report him. He is crazy. He is not a nurse. He's from one of those transitional houses and this is his job training. They gave him a night shift and told him to stay away from the patients. All he is supposed to do is empty the trash." She tells someone to get me a shot for the pain. I tell her I'm tired and just want to be left alone. I don't trust anyone. I can only wonder what she'll inject me with in this mad house.

I get a shot in my hip, the morphine IV drips faster, and the nursing supervisor greets me with a legal pad and report forms. She interrogates me and apologizes, assuring me he will be fired. She's relieved the narcotics have left me somber, speechless, unable to request an attorney. She hopes I'll forget about this incident after the report is filled out and signed, that way he can be fired, and none of this will reflect poorly on her. I don't even care anymore. "I have one favor of you, though," I say before falling asleep. "Could I please be in a new room?"

She's heard the stories about the old woman and assures me something will be done, but there are no empty beds now.

The last thing I hear before falling asleep is my roommate chanting: "Delores finally got what she deserves."

The next morning I hear that my doctor is on the floor. I can finally find out what went wrong and ask when I'll be released. I hear him talking fast into his little recorder, reciting a series of facts for someone to type later.

A nurse comes in and pulls open my curtain. I ask her to keep it closed but she says they're going to move me to another bed while they put clean sheets on mine. They have to wheel it in. As soon as she leaves, my roommate yells, "You're a spoiled brat, Delores!" Without any effort, she throws her water glass and the plastic water bottle at me. She even makes a mistake and throws her dentures. Nothing breaks. It just lands on my leg.

My doctor walks in and sees his expensive surgery being ruined. "I'll sue you for every penny you have if you hurt her," he screams. He bellows in the hallway for someone to remove her now.

The old woman weeps. "Where is my son? He's supposed to take me home." They wheel her away. I hear her endless stream of Delores curses.

"I heard about that man last night," the doctor says. "You're having a bad time here, aren't you?"

"What happened to my leg?" I asked.

"It was worse than I expected," he says. Don't worry, you'll be good as new soon."

"Will I be able to drive?"

"Not for several months."

"But you promised I'd be up and at it in three weeks."

"These things happen," he says, as he pats me on the head, and I know there are at least four more days to be spent in this hospital room.

The nurse turns up my morphine after talking with the doctor in the hallway. I lie in a muddled haze, thinking about how often these things happen.

I drift off to sleep with Mrs. Booth by my side, yelling obscenities and tossing her belongings.

There is no empty room.

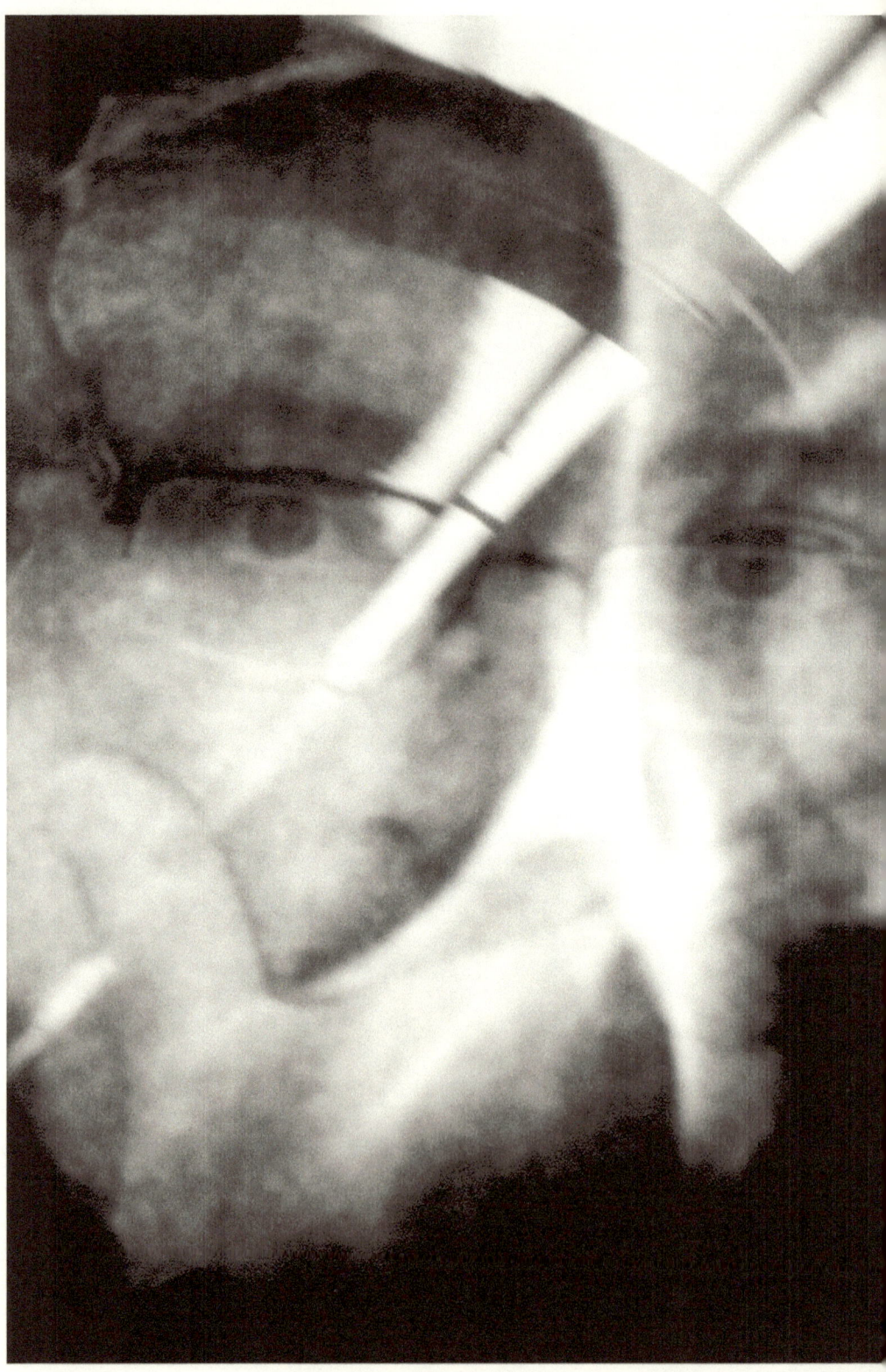

DAVID W. PAGE

BURR HOLES IN THE HEART

burr: a form of drill used for creating openings in skull bone to relieve pressure from intracranial hemorrhage

In the subdued light of the ICU isolation room, Lisa's thirty-one-year-old body hides beneath a single white sheet. Obscene numbers rivet her racing pulse to the overhead monitor. QRS complexes dart after each other across the screen like skittish fireflies. Without warning her blood pressure sags to ninety over sixty. An alarm sounds.

A nurse peeks into Lisa's cubicle. "Should I call a code?"

"Not yet," I say, gambling.

Lisa's breathing deteriorated moments before she was admitted to the ICU when an endotracheal tube was inserted into her throat. She was attached to a ventilator and a surgical consultation was requested for "a question of sepsis." Was the young woman infected? Other than a minor gynecologic procedure a few days earlier, Lisa had no significant past medical history. On-call for our group, that was pretty much the skeleton of her story I received.

So at two in the morning, three days after what turned out to be an elective laparoscopy for pelvic pain, I evaluate Lisa in her dimly lighted cubicle. I receive a tangle of mixed signals—electronic, visual, olfactory, and most important for a surgeon, the palpable truth spoken by rigid abdominal wall muscles, stone-hard stiffness informing my examining hand. In that brief moment at her bedside, I discover her illness is chewing at a lifetime of health, her body shriveling up in the rabid fires of infection.

"They think she's in septic shock," says the night shift nurse, hanging a bag of antibiotics. "She's been like this for most of the day."

"What do they think caused it?" I eye Lisa under the forgiving sheet. Her urine is the color of Killian Red. When I touch her belly again to be certain, Lisa reacts as if shot. Her eyes widen, wrists twist against the woven fabric of her

restraints.

"Something in her belly they think," the nurse said.

Why am I receiving this information second-hand? Because the doctors who asked for the consult are at home in bed and did not extend to me a personal phone call. I probe Lisa's lower abdomen. "Right here?"

Her abdominal muscles tighten. I release the pressure and Lisa's head jerks off the pillow. The breathing tube and its corrugated tubing yank at the corner of her mouth and she falls back on her damp pillow. Lisa's strawberry blond hair streaks her forehead, glued to her sweaty skin in strings. It's called rebound tenderness—proof of peritonitis. I turn away from her dilated gaze with a growing sense of dread. On an overhead shelf the EKG monitor races. I decide quickly, intuitively, faintly hearing a lawyer's voice asking what evidence I used to make the diagnosis. Surgeons surely trip on the dread of the legally possible in moments like this.

I turn back to Lisa and bend over the bed. Her eyes flicker when I introduced myself as a surgeon over the noise of her ventilator and beeping EKG monitor. Knife bites from her fingernails leave marks in my palm, her strength out of proportion to her sickness. And in that compressed moment, I see camouflaged beneath the sheets and bandages and IV bags and the mucous-rattling endotracheal tube, a frightened young woman. For the life of me, I don't remember the color of Lisa's eyes.

Her chart describes a diagnostic laparoscopy days earlier after which she developed urinary retention. She required catheterization. Lisa's fever shot up a day later while she lay in bed at home. Shortly thereafter she suffered the first in a series of teeth-chipping rigors, a spree of shaking chills that terrified her mother and brought Lisa to the Emergency Department gasping for breath. Within an hour of arriving in the ER, Lisa had been transferred to the ICU. Antibiotics and a quest for the source of her infection were begun. An abdominal CT scan identified fluid in her belly. Was it pus? Ask a surgeon.

I meet with Lisa's parents in the early hours of that first morning and explain that their daughter has a life-threatening infection brewing in her abdomen. Lisa needs an emergency operation. They don't seem surprised. Lisa's father looks familiar to me.

The ICU nurses move swiftly. They prep Lisa for surgery. I don't share my reservations about coming to the case late with her parents. They say we surgeons are often intuitive. Well, at that point I already suspect my operation will be too late. And try as I may to think otherwise on the trip to the operating room, I again imagine myself explaining Lisa's death at our weekly Mortality and Morbidity Conference, and quite possibly much later, when sadness ferments into the corn liquor of anger, in court. It is almost impossible not to think these thoughts as dread of a terrible outcome rides side-saddle on the facts.

Lisa clutches my fingers as we push her ICU bed from the intensive care unit down a long hospital corridor to the elevators. A nurse inflates her lungs with an Ambu bag; Lisa's eyes are huge, darting from face to face. An orderly helps me propel the heavy hospital bed across the gap left by the open elevator door. The jolt bounces Lisa's body. She squeezes my fingers like a vice grip.

In the operating room, I place surgical drapes over Lisa's prepped abdominal skin for sterility, and, of course, to keep her humanity out of sight. It is time to shift gears. I must transition hastily from compassionate caregiver, thinking of my own daughter asleep at home, to resolute surgeon. A Himalayan ice crevasse is smaller than the emotional distance surgeons must leap in a heartbeat between empathy and focused indifference. The risks are deadly if you miss your footing.

Lisa's abdomen lies exposed between fat-pouting lips of a midline abdominal incision. My entry is quick, efficient. The surgical resident assisting me is a junior, untested, but observant. The first whiff of putrid air hits us from the open wound. Lisa's blood pressure slithers, unobtainable for a moment. The anesthesiologist mutters something vile.

"Problem?" I ask over the ether screen.

"Pressure's going south," says the anesthesiologist. "I'll bolus her with fluid. Keep going."

I slip a gloved hand into Lisa's belly. "We've got lots of pus down here."

"CT scan was right," says my assistant.

"Apparently."

Youth attuned to the prognostic shadow dance of technology, I find his remark audacious, his infatuation with images distracting him from the vile reality stinking up the room.

Not only did she have putrid fluid inside her abdominal cavity, Lisa's abdominal wall also bulged with foul-smelling pus trapped in sinewy pockets, killing her by inches. I cut into Lisa's belly wall muscles. Creamy infected fluid spurts onto our sterile drapes. The operating room floods with the stench of rotting tissue.

We run two suctions. Ugly sucking noises turn the disciplined dialogue of the anesthesiologist into an incomprehensible mumble. The middle of three laparoscopic incisions—the central stab wound over her bladder—looks inflamed.

It takes less than an hour to explore and irrigate Lisa's abdomen, clean her abdominal wall, close, and transfer her to the post-anesthesia recovery room.

I wash up and change into fresh scrubs. I head toward the waiting room where Lisa's parents await me in morning's ambivalent lull.

What I did not know I had missed at surgery (would not learn for another three or four days when my associate re-explored Lisa), was a tiny hole in her urinary bladder. Later, we surmised the Veress needle (used to inflate the belly cavity during the original laparoscopy) had punctured Lisa's bladder. When a cystogram, an X-ray of her bladder, showed contrast material spilling into her belly, and when cultures of her urine *and* the abdominal pus grew the same nefarious organism, we knew the origin of Lisa's problem: she'd developed a ravenous bladder infection after her diagnostic laparoscopy.

Tragically, the innocent urinary tract infection had been left to rage out of control. As pressure in Lisa's bladder grew, pus escaped through the bladder wall hole, overflowed into her belly and abdominal wall, and caused a picture of generalized sepsis. The raging infection had swiftly marched forward. It caused an unforgiving condition known as systemic inflammatory response syndrome, or SIRS, which quickly transformed into the deadly early stages of multiple organ failure. It was the condition in which I had found Lisa in the ICU when I first examined her—ventilator-dependent, feverish, and with a high white blood count—that had made me suspicious of the inflammatory killer. I was now convinced the process had accelerated out of control like an Australian brush fire *before* I operated on Lisa.

When I performed Lisa's surgery, her inflamed bladder tissues had squeezed the putative puncture hole shut. That's why I had not seen it. The good news: there was no on-going contamination. No more leak. If I had been called sooner, Lisa might have survived.

The family's lawyer didn't see it that way.

When my associate operated on Lisa a week later, he found no further infection, no urine leak, no pus pocket, but he did see the tiny hole in the bladder. Sad days of what seemed like futile treatment crept into Lisa's ICU course. Outlaw bodily responses, buckets of destructive enzymes flooded Lisa's tissues and led to a downward spiral of multiple organ failure that ended her life two weeks after my consultation. In the end, I knew Lisa only by her infected body and the frantic communication we had momentarily shared beside her stretcher on the way to the operating room. I will always remember the terror Lisa's eyes deeded to me when she pleaded for mercy, squeezing my hand that long night.

I sit with Lisa's parents. We are in the ICU waiting room. We stumble cautiously through the first hour of anguish after Lisa's death, thinking out loud about what had happened, waiting to go back into the ICU to say goodbye. We discuss her illness and my conviction that Lisa's immune system had unraveled before my knife found its mark. The process is well described in the scientific literature, I explain. A point in time is reached with raging sepsis when the body's physiology cannot be repaired, the terrible bugs swarm and win, and some molecular critical distance is surpassed. We surgeons say this with conviction, knowing it to be true, almost certainly sounding defensive.

"Hope I don't sound as if I'm making excuses," I tell Lisa's parents. "We call it the 'systemic inflammatory response syndrome,' a snowball effect we can't stop once it starts. It's impossible to know when the line of irreversibility was crossed with your daughter."

Lisa's father seems vaguely convinced, but confused. Her mother shows no reaction to my explanation, her dark eyes wet, uncertain, locked on me, her radar seeking clues. I reword my explanation. This time Lisa's mother asks me if I thought the laparoscopy had anything to do with the infection.

"My associate found a hole in Lisa's bladder," I say. "It played a role."

It is impossible to end a death talk. You sneak around and around on a frightening path, and you see it narrowing up ahead, closing in on the truth with ever smaller explanatory strides until you discover you're staring into your own soul. In the early hours of the morning Lisa died, the unspoken atrocity sullied our conversation: a thirty-one-year-old healthy woman is dead.

The hardware of my surgical intervention, tubes, drains, bandages, even the ventilator, seem like archeological artifacts in Lisa's brief hospital history, the debris of failure her parents see when we stand mute and they say their final farewell in Lisa's curtained room. Nothing I had done had helped Lisa. I had simply been called too late, a slippery reality absent from the medical record.

When her brother appeared in my office, I was stunned. Lisa's parents had never mentioned him. Where was he during the throes of his sister's demise? Where was he when his parents suffered the most profound tragedy of their enjoined lives? What family connections lay hidden from me?

Although I could not answer these queries, I did understand why he sat before me now. It wasn't the threat of litigation that saddened me. The absentee stakeholder, this invisible brother, had the right to keep and bear grudges. And so as he bluntly rehashed his understanding of the facts of Lisa's death, his parents sat next to him and suffered through his queries in silence.

Her brother's insistence that something had gone wrong, that something must have been done incorrectly, negligence in a word, brought back my own sister's death in Canada in 1971. I snapped back to her head-on car collision on a remote Canadian road and a small Ontario hospital's failure to provide the most basic emergency care. Sandy had been transferred to Ottawa General Hospital. She died within an hour of neglected minor injuries and the simple need for IV fluid resuscitation withheld in the northern community hospital. The autopsy report—an impersonal recitation of my adopted sister's organs and tissues—had resided in my bottom desk drawer for years, the residual of a lost family relationship, ammunition for a legal battle I lost the heart to fight, and hidden in a memory-proof container until Lisa's brother pried off the lid.

I experienced shame and anger when Lisa's brother brought me to tears in my own office, remembering Sandy's case, real medical malfeasance. But that wasn't the source of my wet eyes, averted behind tissues before reasserting my game face against his indignity. It was my failed relationship with Sandy that burst my heart that day.

It's called a deposition.

It should be properly referred to as prolonged emotional torture, psychological waterboarding. It was how, a few months later, Lisa's brother extracted his measure of revenge. A clever Boston lawyer worked me over for two hours, drilling random burr holes into my heart, expecting guilt to pour out of my ventricles, seeking an admission of guilt I didn't feel and refused to own. He drilled into my conscience without relieving the pressure and only reluctantly accepting my SIRS explanation of Lisa's demise after hours of interrogation.

The inexorable consequence of neglected sepsis finally became a matter of record. Having failed to indict me with that line of inquiry, the Boston lawyer then attempted to coerce me into incriminating the gynecologist who had performed the laparoscopy. His inquiries felt like electric shocks from alligator clips leading from a car battery and clamped to my conscience.

Eventually, I was released from Lisa's brother's lawsuit without prejudice, but with a lifetime of regret, Lisa's memory evermore glued to my sister Sandy's—two young women who should not have died.

Eventually, I remembered where I'd seen Lisa's father. And so for years we encountered each other at our local professional hockey team's games. He was a goal judge; me, an occasional team doctor. We always shook hands and talked of hockey and other things. I sensed no hostility in his presence. His grasp was forgiving. It reminded me of Lisa's hand clutched in mine that night of failure.

In those greetings, Lisa's father granted me a measure of reprieve from the guilt I still own for having lost his daughter's life, SIRS or not. And I would like to think he understands that in my mind at least the tragedy of Lisa's and my sister's deaths are inseparably linked. Both could have been avoided.

I've seen both sides of loss in my surgeon's years. The burden saddens me. Of course, there are elements of the care we gave Lisa to question, the delay in getting her treated, the poor communication between the gynecologist and me. The healing art often stumbles in the dark when the science underfoot leaves an incompletely cleared path.

The answer is seldom litigation. Punishment leaves scars. And scar tissue retracts into itself. To compassionately manage a treatment catastrophe, one must care for the wounded survivors. Doctors too.

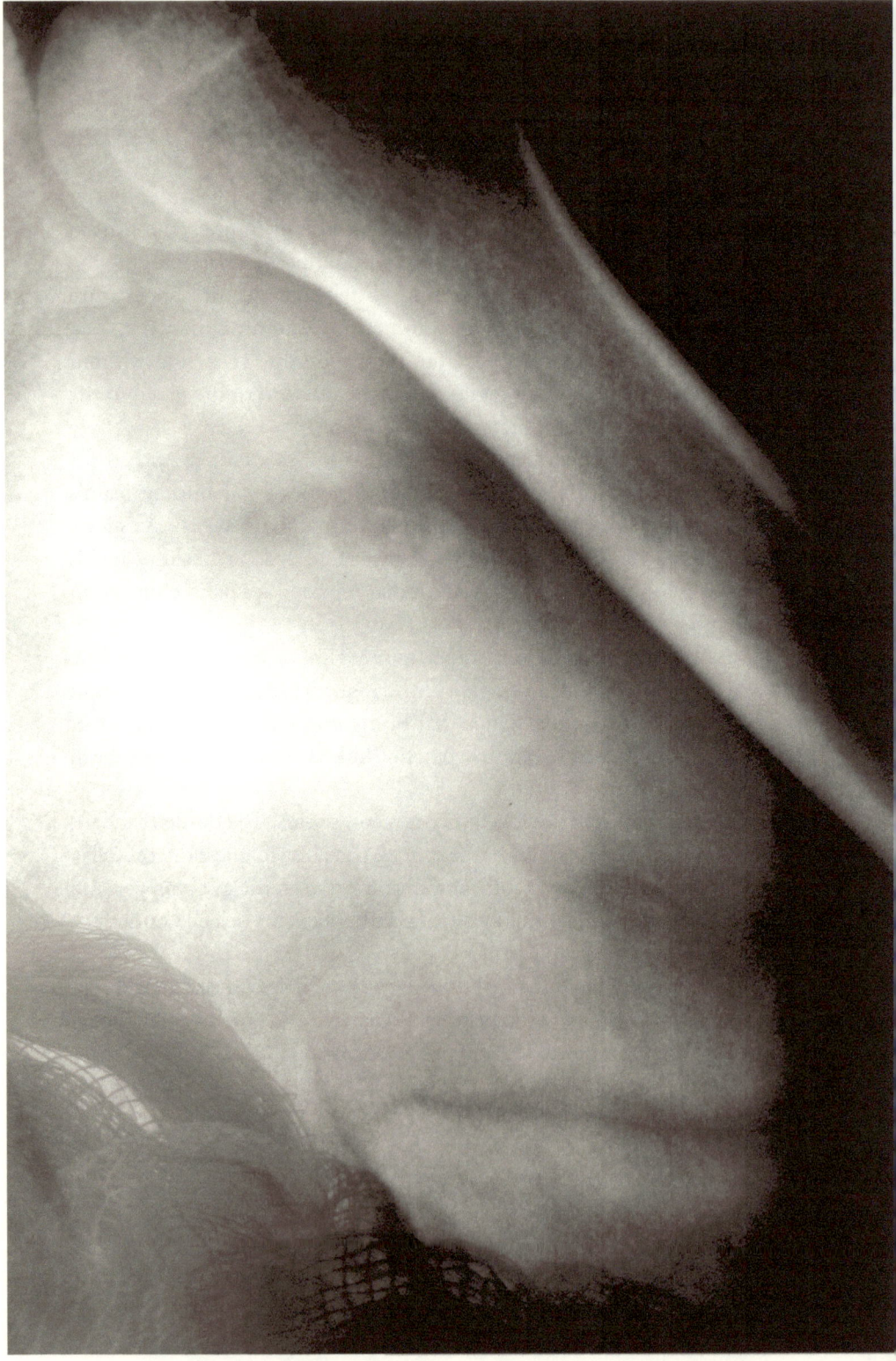

VI
GROWING IN OUR ROLES

ELAINE MORGAN

ZEN AND THE ART OF MEDICAL APPOINTMENTS

Remember the good old days of one doctor for all of your ailments? One kindly neighborhood doctor who knew you, your family, and who took care of all of the paperwork. One familiar face who took the time to listen to what you had to say and who valued your input, knowing that you were the one who was experiencing and he or she was a non-local observer. Well, things have changed, and the term 'team approach' is causing me a lot of time-consuming work, energy and strategy.

In this twenty-first century, I prepare my medical history at home prior to my appointments with my Internist, Rheumatologist, or my Orthopedic doctor. I collate and coordinate all laboratory results, radiology reports and copies of medical letters with findings, depending upon the type of specialist being seen at the time, which part of the body is involved, and what would be considered eye-catching paperwork for each doctor.

If the problem is anatomical, I draw a diagram of the human body, front and back, being careful that it is in freehand and an imperfect artistic endeavor. I do not want to give the doctor the impression that I'm talented artistically as well as intellectually, or that I've taken too much time pondering my anatomy.

I mark all pain areas with a red pen, drawing corresponding lines with factual descriptions of what hurts and how it feels. I always make sure the handwriting is sloppy and the notes are written in simple, layperson's non-medical terminology such as, the small of the back in the butt instead of the lumbar area, the collar bone instead of the clavicle, the butt instead of the gluteal area, and the ribs instead of the costal cartilage.

I read my notes to the doctors during the visit, feigning memory problems with advancing age, and I'm careful to say at strategic points, "I do not understand what the lab results mean. I do not understand what the Radiologist is writing about. I don't understand this medical terminology at all. I'm not a doctor. I can only point to where it hurts. I only copied this from the reports and put this down in my notes because it may be related, but I really don't know for sure."

I'm also careful to act as though getting to the source of the problem was purely accidental and I preface everything I say with statements like, "Gee doctor, do you think there may be a connection here? Do you think there is a relationship between this and that? Gee doctor, it hurts here. Do you think maybe there could be a problem?"

I strive to cultivate a Zen posture, having studied the art of complaining and, at the same time, non-complaining. I smile during the non-complaints, keeping in mind that if I do not I may be viewed as a hypochondriac, a female patient with free-floating Generalized Anxiety Disorder, or as presenting with a flat affect.

I distinguish between acting overly-concerned and getting my point across, the fine line between whining and legitimate complaints, backed up by the written material presented, and the fine line between getting the doctor's attention and eyes focused on the paperwork instead of on the ceiling or on the wall. Also, the fine line between acting dumb when making a suggestion towards the solution and a possible treatment modality. I always let the doctor think the solution has come from his or her own mind and medical acumen. I had to learn this tactic the hard way.

I strive to keep the humor light and seemingly spontaneous, with the wise use of metaphor at the medically correct moments, with the proper and acceptable wince of the eyes, with a whine in the voice at appropriate times (I use this one sparingly) to indicate I'm truly dependent upon the doctor's expertise, even if I have figured it all out by myself before the appointment. I also keep the metaphors simple so the doctor will get it.

Everything I know and present must appear to have been arrived at through accidental means and I always keep in mind there is another fine line between an ostentatious display of gratitude and a humble display, the latter of which is the most popular with the medical profession.

As a physically challenged individual who has been on the 'doctor wheel' for many years, and one who is not a recognized member of her own medical team, I have also learned to prepare myself for all medical appointments by reading the following material beforehand: *The Chinese Art of War* by Sun Tzu, *Book of the Five Rings* by Miyamoto Musachi, and *The Japanese Art of War: Understanding the Culture of Strategy.*

JOHN MANESIS

WEN

The first time we made rounds
as junior medical students
at the Omaha V.A. Hospital,
we crowded behind Dr. Kleitch,
a handful of foot soldiers
in the company of a General.
The conversations on the ward
came to a halt in mid-sentence
as he made his entrance,
a compact surgeon with grey hair
that bristled, wire rimmed glasses
and eyes glinting like ball bearings.
He stopped to examine a patient
who dangled his feet over the bedside.
Dr. Kleitch pointed to a lump
on the man's forehead and asked me,
"What's that, Doctor?"
I stared at the swelling,
hoping in vain it would somehow
reveal its mysteries to me,
and replied, "I don't know."
"You don't know? I am sure even
he knows," the surgeon proclaimed,
glaring at the patient who gulped,
cleared his throat and said,
"Sorry, me neither, Doc."
I thought I saw a faint smile
trying to escape from the corner
of our leader's mouth.

"It's a wen . . . spelled, W..E..N,
a sebacious cyst, Doctors,
benign, well circumscribed,
non-tender, soft, and commonly seen
on the face, scalp or back.
Don't ever forget it!"
I survived that initiation,
my boot camp, with a flesh wound
but no internal injuries.
To this day, whenever I see a wen,
the curtains of the past part,
Dr. Kleitch strides onto the stage
and there I am in the front row,
lucky to have a ticket to the show.

ROBERT P. STICCA

THIS GUY MIGHT MAKE IT

The sound of the pager pierced through the fog of a deep sleep, waking me with a start. Beep, Beep, Beep—Beep, Beep, Beep. *Is that the trauma page?* Can't be—the hospital is supposed to be on diversion because of the nursing strike. Must be dreaming.

BEEP, BEEP, BEEP—BEEP, BEEP, BEEP.

It's the trauma page. Better wake up, better answer it quick. More by reflex than deliberate action, I snapped the light on and pressed the button on the pager. The clock read 2:15 a.m. A disconcerting message showed on the digital window of the pager: 5295*1. I recognized the number. A stat page to the ER.

Shit. This hospital is supposed to be closed. Why did the paramedics bring the patient here?

5295, 5295. I'd only seen the numbers for a fraction of a second, but it was as if I had known them my whole life as I fumbled for the phone and dialed.

"ER, Janie Stewart."

"Hello, this is Dr. Sticca. What's going on?"

"The ambulance is arriving now. Thirty-six-year-old black male involved in an altercation in a bar, stab wound to the right chest. He's in bad shape. Blood everywhere. BP very low. Barely alive."

"Why did they bring him here?"

"They didn't think they could make it to another hospital. It happened just a few blocks away."

"Have you called the chief resident? "

"He's not in the hospital. Because of the strike, they let all the senior residents go home. You're the only surgical resident here."

Shit. Shit. Double Shit. "OK, I'll be right there." Jesus Christ. I'm only a second-year resident; I can't handle something like this. Where are my shoes? Where's my lab coat? No time to wash up or brush my teeth; got to get there, ASAP.

This wasn't supposed to happen. It was supposed to be an easy day—staying in-house for call was only a formality, due to the strike. While the rotation at Carney Hospital in the Dorchester section of Boston was liked and eagerly anticipated by the Boston University surgery residents, the nursing strike had put a damper on the rotation. Surgical residents live by the dictum "A chance to cut is a chance to cure." Whenever the chance to cut was not present, the surgical residents' interests waned quickly.

The nursing union had declared a strike about a week ago and the hospital was limited to a few very basic functions without nursing staff to care for the patients. Only two of eighteen operating rooms were functioning, and there were very few inpatients. Elective surgeries were all cancelled. The surgical residents couldn't wait for the end of the strike, but secretly, the relief from the grind of working over a hundred hours per week was welcomed—at least for the first week.

It had been an easy day for the second-year surgery residents, starting with rounds at 5 a.m. Although there were no surgeries scheduled, the routine for early morning rounds was so engrained that it was hard to break. After rounds and taking care of the few remaining inpatients in the morning, a noon teaching conference and outpatient clinic in the afternoon, the residents that were not on call went home. Since these activities did not have to be worked in between the usual elective surgeries, the day ended several hours shorter than the standard twelve-to-fourteen hour days. (In 1985, mandatory eighty-hour workweek maximums for physicians-in-training did not exist.) During the strike, the residents actually arrived home by 5 p.m. Our wives and children didn't know what to make of it.

General surgery has long been viewed as the toughest of all specialties to train in. Originally designed by Dr. William Halsted, the father of American surgery, in the early nineteenth century, the training has changed little since then. The five years are the longest of any specialty for basic training. Nowadays, as many as seventy percent of surgical residents go on to train in a surgical subspecialty for another two to three years, extending the rigors of training even longer. Viewed as masochists by other trainees in medicine, surgeons take a perverse pleasure in knowing that they are expected to work the hardest and have the most difficult hours of any residency in medicine.

Every medical student has to make a decision as to what specialty he/she will spend the rest of his/her life practicing by the end of the third year of medical school. This is probably not the best time, as by the end of the third year each student has only had a short time to experience the major specialties in medicine: pediatrics, obstetrics and gynecology, surgery, psychiatry, internal medicine, and family practice. Because the application and interview process for specialty training occurs during the fourth year of medical school, this decision must be made by the end of the third year.

For me, this decision was more difficult than most. I had started medical school a few years later than the standard age of twenty-two. I was married the year before I began medical school and my son, our first child, was born while I was a third-year medical student. Before doing my surgical rotation, I was aware of its grueling work hours, so surgery was not initially a consideration for me. I didn't think I could bear to be away from my growing family.

But a strange thing happened during my surgery rotation. I fell in love with it. The surgical mentality, the hard work, and the ability to cure a disease process with an operation all appealed to my persona. This, coupled with comments from my surgical preceptors on my better-than-average technical abilities, gave me cause to reconsider my previous plans. After many long discussions with my wife, I realized that I would not be happy in another specialty. Her consent and encouragement was the last bit of evidence I needed to pursue a career in surgery. Despite these convictions, there were lingering doubts about this choice. Could I do it? Would the training be too tough for me and my family? Would I be able to do what was necessary in an emergency situation? I loved the work, but the 120-hour workweeks only reinforced my uncertainty.

There is a well-defined caste system in surgical training. Each year of training brings on different levels of technical tasks and patient care responsibilities. As the lowest members of the team, interns or first-year residents take care of the pre- and postoperative patients, seeing them daily, gathering lab and X-ray reports, writing notes, and doing other menial tasks or "scut" work. Their operative experience consists of easier cases— appendectomies and hernia repairs—but even then they are at the mercy of the chief resident, who may or may not assign these cases to the wanting intern. Each year, if the resident is fortunate enough to get promoted to the next level of training, the degree of responsibility and difficulty of surgical cases increases.

The fifth-year chief resident controls most aspects of the surgical service, including distributing the workload, assigning the surgical cases, and making the call schedule. In addition, the chief supervises and teaches all residents below him and is ultimately responsible for all aspects of the surgery team. This responsibility can be a heavy weight to bear, often making the chief cranky and irritable. The chief resident can make the junior residents' lives a living hell or a fantastic experience, all depending on his/her personality, sense of fairness and organizational ability. All surgical trainees, including the chief resident, are supervised by attending surgeons who have completed their surgical training, but there is an unwritten rule that the attendings will rarely interfere with the chief resident's authority over the junior residents.

The ER was about a five-minute walk from the call rooms. I made it in about sixty seconds by running down the five flights of stairs two at a time, a trick I learned from Charlie Eaton, a chief resident who I actually liked and respected.

Upon arriving in the ER trauma room, the scene was chaos. The receptionist's description was accurate—there was blood everywhere. It seemed to be coming from a gaping stab wound in the right axilla (armpit), which had obviously lacerated the major artery and vein running from the heart to the right arm. The victim was unconscious and barely breathing, his blood pressure was low—in fact, barely obtainable.

The nursing staff all looked up when I entered the room, waiting for someone, usually the chief resident, to take charge. As a second-year resident, I did not have the experience or training to take this type of responsibility. But there was no one else to do it. With the hospital closed, there were no other surgeons around to take over. The patient would be dead in a matter of seconds. His heart rate was already slowing, indicating an impending cardiac arrest. Sure, I had seen and assisted on a few traumas as an intern at Boston

City Hospital, but that was different. There was always someone else there to take the responsibility and give the orders. At Boston City, all I had to do was obey orders, watch and learn. Now it was *me* in charge, with no one to pass the buck to. But there was nothing to lose. In a minute or two this patient would be dead, unless something was done, and quick.

What's first? The ABC's of trauma, a sequence that is pounded into a surgical resident's brain a thousand times: Airway, Breathing, Circulation. Find an airway to get oxygen to the lungs first, or everything else will be useless. Without oxygen in the lungs to get absorbed into the blood stream and circulated to the vital organs, life is not sustainable.

No difficult thought process here. An unconscious patient who is not breathing adequately—intubate him and put him on a ventilator.

"Nurse, where's the intubation tray."

"Right here, doctor. Which blade do you want?"

"I will take the straight Miller blade. Can someone extend the neck?"

As I pried open the mouth, a rush of vomitus was expelled. I was ready to vomit myself. "Great, OK, I need the suction, quick."

With rapid suctioning, I was able to clear the airway, but even then there was no spontaneous respiratory activity. I knew that he needed to be intubated. I had practiced intubation on a manikin many times, but this was different. Manikins didn't have French fries in their throat. Manikins didn't die if you couldn't get the tube in. After clearing the airway, I was actually able to see the vocal cords, a critical step in getting the tube in the right place. Even more surprisingly, the tube slid into place in the trachea without difficulty.

"OK, I think the tube is in the right place, can someone listen to the lungs for breath sounds?"

"It sounds good, doctor," the nursing staff said, and I sensed a new tone of respect.

"OK, connect the tube to the vent, use these settings—Rate-16, O_2-100%, PEEP-5."

Maybe I can do this. OK, what's next? Airway—OK—the tube is in good place. Breathing—OK—the patient is now on the ventilator and has good respirations. Circulation—major problem.

"Nurse, can you tell me what the blood pressure is?"

"Doctor, we can't get a blood pressure."

The monitor revealed that there was still electrical activity in the heart, but there was little or no blood in it. Hemorrhagic shock is an interesting phenomenon. If there is massive blood loss and the heart has no fluid to pump to the vital organs, everything stops. This patient was in the worst stage of hemorrhagic shock. He had probably lost 75 percent of his blood volume and didn't have enough blood in his vascular system to keep the circulation going. He needed fluid, lots of fluid.

"How much fluid has he gotten?"

"None, doctor. We can't get an IV, his veins are all collapsed. We've tried several sites."

"OK, no blood pressure, I guess we should start chest compressions. I need to get some IV lines started, and fast. Do you have a cutdown kit?"

"Yes, Doctor, right here"

"Open it. Quickly." I tried to act calm. If ever there was a need for Nam lines, this was it. I had heard and read about 'Nam' lines several times. This was a rapid and crude form of an IV that could be used to give large volumes of fluid in seconds. They were first described in the Vietnam War when badly wounded soldiers in hemorrhagic shock needed rapid infusions of large volumes of fluid and blood. The concept is simple. Place the largest tube possible in the most accessible vein that can accommodate it, and then use it to give the fluid and blood as quickly as possible. In Vietnam they had discovered that it was a waste of time to fool around with the standard intravenous catheters to give these volumes of fluid. The IV catheters were so small that they only served as a bottleneck for the large volumes of fluid that were needed. These IVs were fine for the usual fluid volumes that were given, approximately 100-200 cc/hour, but when giving 100-200 cc/*minute*, they couldn't handle it.

Basic fluid mechanics says that the larger the diameter of the tube, the more fluid that can flow through it. The solution reached in Vietnam was to use the IV tubing directly, which was at least ten times larger than even the largest IV catheter. The tubing was cut tangentially and inserted directly into the saphenous vein, a large vein just under the skin of the inner aspect of the thigh. With a little practice, these could be placed in thirty to sixty seconds. I had only seen this done once before at Boston City. I didn't have time to practice.

"I'm going to put Nam lines in," I said hesitantly.

Eyebrows raised. There were several questioning glances around the room. There weren't many alternatives. The patient was dying in front of us, for lack of fluid volume.

"OK, doctor, tell us what you need."

"Get that IV tubing over here and hook it to a large bag of normal saline." As I slashed the inner aspect of the thigh with the scalpel, I prayed that the saphenous vein would be where it was in the anatomy books. A brief moment of dissection, and Yes, there it was. A quick incision into the vein and insertion of the tube and the fluid was running in. 500 cc in about two minutes—great. The second Nam line in the other leg was even quicker. With two Nam lines, both fluid and blood could be given rapidly.

"Doctor, we have a blood pressure of 70 systolic, and the heart rate is down to 120."

"Great, give two units of O negative blood and keep the normal saline running in as fast as possible." *OK, now we're cooking with gas. This guy might make it.* The blood pressure was coming up and the heart was now pumping efficiently. He had only been about two to three minutes without adequate circulation, not enough to cause brain death, but it was impossible to tell until the patient was stabilized and woke up. In most circumstances, the human brain can tolerate up to four to six minutes of poor blood flow without permanent damage. I hoped that the critical time for brain injury had not been reached.

"What's the blood pressure now?"

"90/60 but we have a problem."

"What?"

"Look at his axilla, there's blood gushing out all over."

Right—the injury that had caused all of this was still there. While the patient was in hemorrhagic shock without any circulation, no blood came from the lacerated blood vessels in the axilla. But now that circulation had been restored, the spickets were open again and the blood was pouring out.

I pointed to one of the young orderlies, watching in awe. "Joe, come here, get some gloves on. Grab these sterile towels and put pressure under the arm, here." Most bleeding can be stopped with direct pressure, and this situation was no different. With pressure on the lacerated blood vessels in the axilla, and fluid infusing, the blood pressure and pulse began to normalize. *This guy can make it!* There still were a lot of hurdles to get over: he could develop organ failure, he might have brain damage. But he was doing better, and we were doing everything we could.

"OK, call the OR, tell them to get ready because we're coming up. Has anybody called Dr. Carroll and the chief resident? Who's the chief on call tonight? Rob Grasberger. OK, get him on the phone. Joe, keep pressure on those vessels." It was getting easier to give orders. And surprisingly, people were listening. This was getting better by the minute.

"Doctor Sticca, we have Doctor Grasberger on the phone. Can you talk with him?"

My hands were covered in blood, and I couldn't stop to hold the phone. "Yes, hold the phone to my ear." I told Rob the situation. He was a good chief resident. Not only would he pitch in and help when the shit hit the fan, he wasn't overly impressed with himself and would spend time teaching and guiding the junior residents, as a chief resident should. "We put some Nam lines in and he now has a reasonable blood pressure and pulse. He's still actively hemorrhaging from the axilla. We're controlling it with direct pressure, but this guy needs to go to the OR."

"You put Nam lines in?" Rob said with some incredulity.

"Yeah, he was ready to code, I had no other choice. He's doing better now. Blood pressure 110/60, heart rate—110. We've given him eight liters of saline and four units of blood. I thought this guy was dead when I first saw him, but now I think he might make it."

"Does he have any brain function?"

"Can't tell right now. He was comatose when he came in. He was severely hypotensive only for about three minutes. His pupils are reactive but he hasn't woken up. We've sedated him now, for the OR."

"OK, I'll be there in ten minutes. Is Mitch Carroll coming in?" Dr. Carroll was the chief of surgery, also the attending surgeon on call that night and the one to make the final decision to operate. The chief resident could call him Mitch. I referred to him as Dr. Carroll.

"Yeah, they have called him. I think he is coming in. Do you want me to call him?"

Usually the chief was the one to communicate directly with the attending surgeon, especially for important decisions such as this.

"No, I'll call him. Meet you in the OR."

The situation had calmed down a little in the ER trauma suite. With a stable pulse and blood pressure, I could take a deep breath and try to relax a little. I was still a little shaky, but the patient was doing better, the trauma team was working well together, and I was rapidly adjusting to the role of the team leader. "OK, have the labs come back? We need to get this guy packaged up and into the OR. Has anyone heard from Dr. Carroll? Joe, are you OK? Are you keeping pressure on the bleeding vessels?"

By the time we got to the OR, the entire team was there: Dr. Carroll, Rob Grasberger, the anesthesiologist, and the nursing staff and scrub tech. When the patient arrived, they took over, and I was again relegated to the role of a second-year resident.

And that was OK. It took me some time to realize the magnitude of the last half hour's events. We may have saved a life. *I used some of the knowledge from over five years of studying and training to actually save someone's life!* The hard work, the sleepless nights . . . they had finally made a difference. It felt good, very good.

I was right about the injury. The knife had lacerated the axillary artery and vein. Both of these could be repaired, which took about two hours in the operating room. I watched and assisted as Rob and Dr. Carroll performed the repair. Fortunately, the closely adjacent axillary nerves, which control the function of the arm, were not injured. With blood flow reestablished, the patient would likely recover with intact function of his arm and hand. By 6 a.m. the patient was in the Intensive Care Unit, recovering from surgery.

As we were leaving the OR, Rob Grasberger and Dr. Mitchell asked me about the events in the emergency room. I recounted them in more detail, explaining my trepidations during the resuscitation in the ER, but they both felt that the management had been appropriate for the situation. In fact, they were actually impressed.

"This guy is lucky you were there," said Dr. Carroll.

Heady stuff for a second-year resident. At some time during their training almost every surgical resident experiences doubts and feelings of inadequacy about his/her future ability to function as a surgeon, especially in emergency life or death situations. Mine were fading quickly.

Although I had only two hours of sleep in the past thirty-six hours, fatigue was not an issue. I was still riding an adrenaline high from the emergency room. I spent the morning in the ICU with my patient, monitoring his progress and waiting for signs of brain function. If he woke up and demonstrated higher-level brain function, he would make a complete recovery. This could take days, or even weeks, after an episode of shock.

Later that morning I spoke with the police investigating the incident. I found out that my patient was an accountant who was at a local dance bar and was mistaken for another man who was involved with the assailant's girlfriend. He was attacked with a switchblade in the low lighting of the dance floor. The drunken assailant had been found and arrested. In my limited experience with trauma, I had noticed that almost always, drugs, alcohol or women were involved. This case was no different. I spoke with my patient's family: decent people, and very concerned. I explained the injury to them and the possibility of brain injury. They understood that at that point, it was a waiting game.

Word had spread around the hospital quickly through the ever-present gossip trail. People who I didn't even know viewed me with a new sense of respect, and several approached me in the ICU congratulating me on a job well done. I tried to minimize my part, not knowing if the ultimate outcome would be good.

A little after 1 p.m., the patient started to wake up. He first moved his extremities, then began to open his eyes. In another hour or two, he was able to nod yes or no to questions. My heart raced. *This guy WILL make it!* He was even able to move his right arm and hand—he would recover completely. Both his family and I were ecstatic.

When I finally left the hospital around 7 p.m. that day, my patient was stable and improving every hour. I took a deep breath of fresh air, squinting in the sunlight. Sunlight, not something a surgical resident experiences very often. The drive home was only fifteen minutes, but I was beginning to feel the effects of the continuous high level of activity over the last two days with little rest. As usual, I had missed dinner with my wife and children, but the microwaved leftovers were still good. The kids climbed up on my lap as I sat in the living room, and despite having my one and three-year-old playing on my lap, the exhaustion coupled with a full stomach was too much.

As I drifted off to sleep, I was feeling pretty good. My patient was recovering in the ICU, and it was because of my ability to use my training and skills to help my fellow man. Maybe it wouldn't always be this way, but right then, the euphoria was intoxicating. Maybe I had made the right decision to become a surgeon.

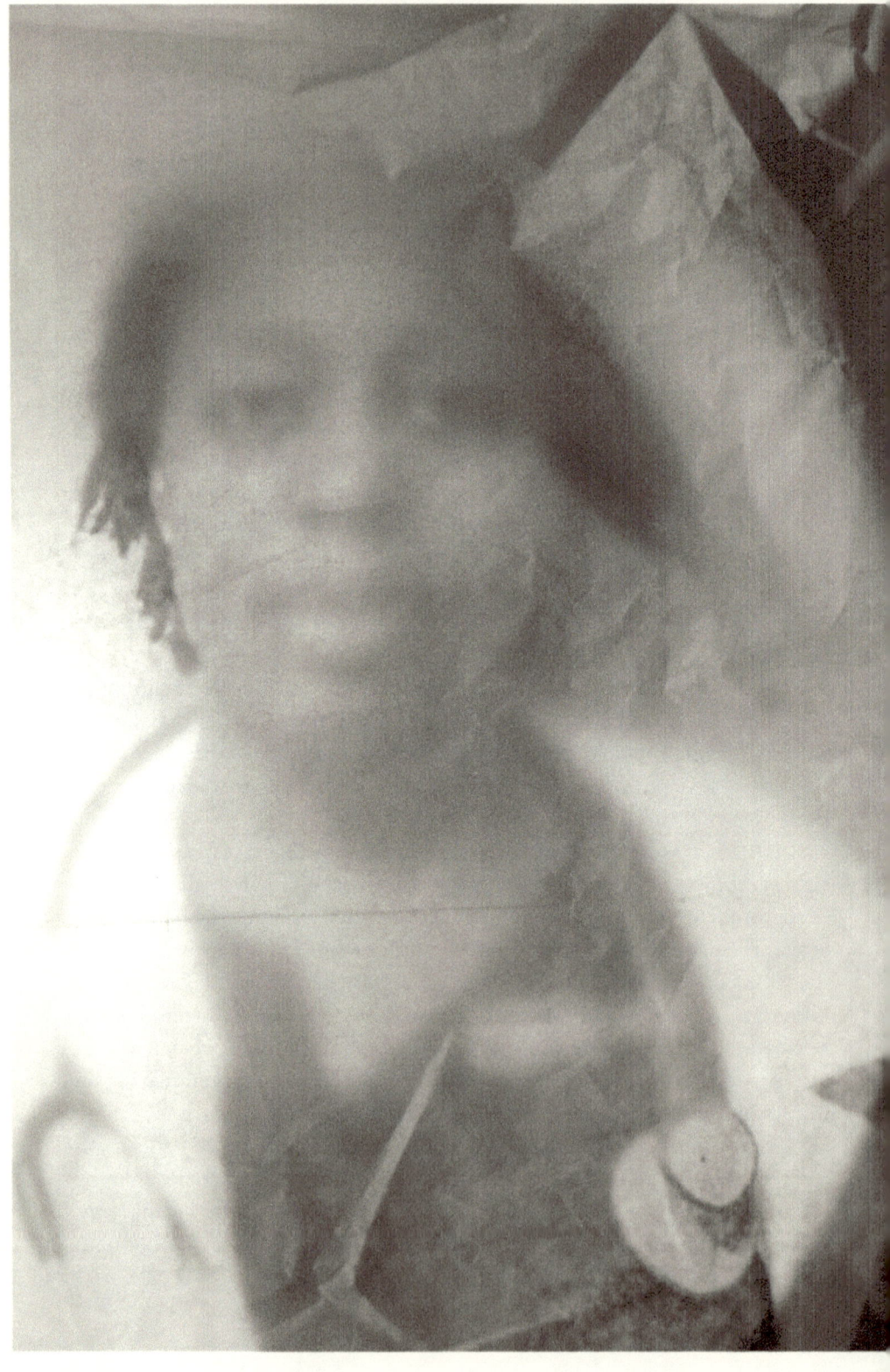

MAXINE SUSMAN

LATE NIGHT HOUSE CALL, PHILADELPHIA, 1938

Lost, somewhere in blocks of rundown walk-ups.
She ducks into Angelo's Bar and Grille,
stethoscope around her neck for protection.
Beer, sweat, sawdust. Dim, stubbled faces
look up at her, woman entering from the dark,

but the bartender knows the street
scribbled on hospital stationery,
someone recognizes the family name,
they send her outfitted with directions
back to the tenements shrouded in rain.

She thinks of relatives left back in Brooklyn,
then of what it will be like to climb
three flights and ring the doorbell

of strangers, to treat a woman in bed
twice her age she's never met
who speaks no English and is in pain.

PATRICIA BARONE

THE HALO CAST

The first time Calla Coffey saw the elderly woman in a halo cast, she wanted to turn on her thick rubber heels and run. It was a horizontal double halo, one metal hoop within the other, with four metal radii coming from the circumference like spokes on a wheel, and fastened through the fine white hair into her skull. Despite being fixed in bone, the halo seemed to float on level with her eyebrows. It was fastened with vertical rods to a neck brace and chest harness that kept her head and neck immobile.

Although her patient could hardly look away from her, Calla liked the way she made eye contact, as if she saw her as a real person, not just hospital staff.

"I'm Calla, your student nurse. Should I call you Mrs. Loom or Zandra?"

"You can call me Mrs. Loom." But she smiled at Calla, not like Mona Lisa because the smile didn't touch the corners of her eyes, but as if she registered an absence of pain, as if smiling didn't hurt this time. "I was flipped onto my neck and head off the hood of a hit-and-run car," she said, as if to get it over with.

She was dressed in a deep blue robe, and Calla wondered how on earth she could help her change her clothes without removing the harness. If she removed the harness improperly, then she might cause harm to the cervical vertebrae. That was some halo cast if it gave two people a headache at the same time.

Because of her graying hair, Calla expected to be questioned when she said student. No one ever commented, and she almost wished that someone would. She wanted to tell someone why she'd decided to try for a better salary, more security, with the result that she had less security. If she could explain it to someone, maybe she'd understand it herself. It was the second week of Calla's last clinical rotation in practical nursing, and she had five more days to go. During this final clinical, the student nurse was supposed to demonstrate that she had it all together, but already she'd made two mistakes. At the Frontenac Technical College, it was three strikes and you're out.

She hadn't almost killed a patient. The first mistake was a medications error. It happened when she'd felt high on her freedom from the close supervision of the instructor. She had busily consulted the pharmacist and Sue, her staff nurse (who was also assigned Calla's patients) about an innocuous antacid medication to be given as needed. The problem was that the doctor had failed to give administration time guidelines.

"You can give these four times in twenty-four hours," Sue said. "Don't bother the doc—they hate that! He'll clarify the order when he makes rounds tomorrow morning."

Not long after Calla gave the medication her instructor tapped on the glass of the chart room. For an instant, as Calla rose, she saw her own face in the glass, her olive skin and black hair superimposed upon and darkening the face of the instructor, who was fair haired and thinner. The instructor closed her eyes for a moment before pronouncing the verdict. "Weren't you taught to never give a medication unless you had the correct time?"

"Yes, I was," Calla said, "I was wrong. I forgot I was a student."

The instructor shook her head. She didn't like the implication that, out in the real world, it was okay for Calla to think for herself that way.

"If your primary nurse wanted to give the med, okay, but you should have said you didn't feel comfortable."

The problem was—she had felt comfortable. All along, all along there've been incidents and accidents (Paul Simon's song an endless loop in her brain), hints and allegations. Things she should know, although she hasn't been taught those things precisely.

The second mistake happened when her patient was taken off to physical therapy before she gave his inhaler. "Don't worry," Sue told her, "you can give it when he gets back." Nonetheless, Calla chased him down to P.T. because she'd been taught that every medication had to be given within one half hour of the time the doctor ordered it. The therapist had her patient in the whirlpool, so Calla waited. It was her lunch half-hour, but she took the old man's chart off the cart to catch up with her charting. At noon, he was still with the physical therapist, and Calla had meds to pass upstairs. So she left, feeling it was better to be damned for one mistake than six.

Fifteen minutes later her instructor arrived pushing Calla's patient in a wheelchair. The patient, an elderly man who had done nothing but complain about having a student, was grinning, and the instructor had a smile clamped to the corners of her lips. Both of their heads were turned toward Calla, who was late on a med and had stranded her patient.

The head of the bed raised automatically and at the same speed—too fast. Only a faint wince on Mrs. Loom's perfectly oval face, a shivering of fine wrinkles. She couldn't have her head raised more than thirty degrees, and Calla double-checked before she wrung out the washcloth and washed her legs, her skin, so papery fine that the terry cloth seemed too rough. It occurred to Calla that she'd seen her at the library, perhaps many times.

When she was a library aide she loved the books, except for Darby Coffey's intrusions. A year ago, when Darby was fired from the tenth job he'd had since they married, he had time to sprawl in the reading room of the library, looking at her with a sneer or scowl. Just when she'd brace herself to refuse to buy him lunch, he'd leave without a backward look. At the safe house, an advocate said, "get him out of the apartment, not you!" Calla collected evidence in a diary, but her fresh black eye did it for the judge, and they served him when he picked up his welfare check. She should have been relieved, but she knew he'd violate the order. He knew where she was at the library, so she quit her job. A student loan just had to tide her over and a loan from the boldest of her three old aunts.

The aunts already had Calla's nurse picture in the Carrio family album: white dress and prim French twist. Aunt Elana was particularly disappointed about the disappearance of the nurse's cap. "It got in the way," Calla said, but she was disappointed too. As if a winged cap would have conferred nursliness.

Mrs. Loom was distant, not much like the aunts, who were bosomy and wept over soap operas. Calla returned with warmer water to finish her bed bath. It was hard to move in these hospital rooms. The wallpaper was the ocher of old contusions, and the walls, exuding a faint smell of antiseptic, pressed in upon the furniture.

Mrs. Loom's shelf had a cactus with purple flowers and a large sculpture: a jade (it couldn't be real!) mountain peak, bonsai trees on the tree line. Close to the top was a tiny hut and smaller human figure, peering out the door at the highest peak, as if wondering about the weather.

"My mountain—the air is thin up there." Mrs. Loom made a grating sound in her throat, and Calla realized that she'd made a joke; it was too late to laugh, so she smiled. "I dislike knick knacks, so she gave me the Himalayas," Mrs. Loom said. "That was my daughter's idea of a prank."

"Your daughter, does she . . ."

"She's dead," Mrs. Loom said, "of cancer, last spring."

"Mrs. Loom was in the news," Sue said. "Struck by a car while she walked in a counter-demonstration outside Planned Parenthood." In the clipping on the nurses' station bulletin board, the straggling line of protesting women were mostly dressed in down jackets except for Mrs. Loom, who wore a long black coat with a hood. Her face in the picture—high cheekbones all bone, the darkness in the sockets of her deep-set eyes—looked even older than she was.

"She's too old to be a woman's libber," Sue said.

"How old is that?" Calla asked. Every now and again, when she had an emotion other than fearful vigilance, she could see that nursing might be fun.

"Oh, you know—over fifty."

Sue was barely thirty. Calla, who was fifty-two, only smiled. She had mixed feelings about abortion. The Carrio sisters, all childless but Calla's mom, rest her soul, said women should make up their own minds, thank you very much, not men and the government! Calla agreed, but, childless as well, she thought of herself as a natural mother. If she and Darby had been able to have children, would things have been better or much worse?

Looking up at the ceiling, Mrs. Loom told Calla about her life. Not like confiding—it was more like overhearing her thoughts. "Seems just yesterday," Mrs. Loom said, her voice weak, as if through a narrowing in her throat. "My husband and I were looking at the last of our babies through the glass in the nursery, and then—in the glass—I'm seeing him walk onto the elevator. Now I can't remember when we divorced. That was the divorce for me."

"How terrible for you!" Calla said. "What a time for him to leave you!"

"He didn't want us to have the last child. I was forty-one. Still, my ex-husband was happier about having a big family than I was. Except for that last baby, my only daughter, and she would be my greatest—well, that's another story. I often wonder, if they'd had safe and legal abortion then, what my life would have been."

"Oh!" Calla flushed up to her forehead. "But you wouldn't wish your children not to have been born?"

"That doesn't enter in. It would have been an alternate life, you see, and I wouldn't have been their mother. If they had to be born, they would have been born to someone else."

Mrs. Loom's face showed no emotion that Calla could recognize. Mrs. Loom was waiting without expectation—did it feel like limbo? Or was that heaven—above your pain at last? Calla felt bruised from the inside with feelings.

"Do you have pain?" Calla asked again as she cleaned the last pin site, halo anchored in bone. Mrs. Loom mouthed "No," but Calla knew that she was lying because she wouldn't take anything for pain except an occasional Tylenol, though she seemed to hurt if she even wrinkled her forehead.

Alternate Lives. Nursing was another life Calla had strayed into. Sometimes she observed herself being a nurse. Who was real—the nurse or the one who watched? No bruises left on Calla's face or arm, her hand holding the cotton tip swab. Darby's hand was so fast it was back to his glass of Killian Red by the time she touched the swelling. You look like that, you get the back of my hand!

Calla shook her head, shaking Darby out. "Mrs. Loom, I'm concerned about the lack of stimulation for you. You don't seem to like television. I bet you're quite a reader."

"For many years, I preferred reading to thinking, but I didn't know that. I thought reading and thinking were the same thing."

Calla turned her just a fraction, keeping one hand on the halo cast. Reading was more like feeling for Calla. The library books used to make her feel enclosed, all the alternative lives in novels and safe to open.

    After lunch, Calla walked past the nursery. A baby's mouth so wide its cheeks swallowed the eyes. In the glass, a ghost woman, her full lips a thin line. How did she look before he hit her? She'd cut her lunch break short to get some reading aides for Mrs. Loom, a book holder and a mirror and magnifying glass that reflected the page up to immobile patients. Mrs. Loom said, "No, I won't read, but thank you for your enterprise." Biting off her words, and Calla felt rebuffed. "I'm in another place, Calla," Mrs. Loom said, as Calla was about to leave. "So are you." It was the first time she'd called her by name, and Calla felt shy, pleased. Had she indeed seen her at the library? She had.

    After taking her noon meds, Mrs. Loom said, "I'm sorry if I seemed abrupt after your thoughtfulness, but all my former lives are just at the edge of my vision. That reading glass—it reminded me of that sign on rear view mirrors—objects are closer than they appear. Reading would make me feel crowded. Do you see?"

    Calla nodded, though she didn't quite see. Time bumped at her white-sleeved elbow. When they took away the date stamp at the library for a bar code scanner, she'd read until someone came through the line and she moved the spines of books across the glass. Books and time flowed past. Now she crammed tasks into the minutes on her neat work sheet, no room for the kinked drainage line, beeping I.V. Calla, crowded by the present. Mrs. Loom, crowded by her past—so much behind her that she had to wait for it to catch up to her.

    As she waited, the elderly woman moved from dreaming to waking and back again, but what she reported to Calla wasn't like a dream though it seemed to come from the same nonlinear source. As Mrs. Loom opened her eyes one morning, she said, "Even people you love the most, they live in their own spheres—like those miniature houses that get snowed on when you turn the globe upside down."

    Here she was, Calla thought, giving intimate help within another person's glass sphere, just that fragile.

    While Calla was setting up an IV for the patient in the next bed, the patient asked Mrs. Loom if she had any grandchildren. "No. One son is gay, another's sterile from a mumps infection, and the oldest is unlikely to marry at this late date."

When her roommate was wheeled out to the visitor's room, Mrs. Loom told Calla that she was trying to think of her daughter's death as a snowstorm in a glass ball. "I can have sun in mine if I choose," she said, her voice so light and even, not breathless but produced without breath. Her head was lifted by the halo cast, even from the softness of the pillow.

Every hospital room looked like every other one until you looked out the window. Calla paused to look out at the frozen marsh bordering the parking lot. At the edge of the wetlands, a fringe of snow fell. How strange, Calla thought, a snow shower. Madonna of the winter fields, wisps of snow in the furrows, her halo worn down like a crescent moon.

On the fourth day of Calla's final clinical, the sky was leaking snow. It had been gray for weeks, the clouds so low and close it was almost as dark at three-thirty, when her shift was over, as it was at six a.m. when she arrived, her white sup-hosed legs tingling from the cold, the nurses passing her like they owned the place, laughing, joking, one with Christmas tree earrings. Instead of taking the elevator to her floor, Calla turned into the coffee shop. I have a right to some private comforts, she decided.

While the night shift nurses were finishing up, Calla called the pharmacy; one of Mrs. Loom's meds was missing. She scanned the lab reports. Loom's potassium was just below normal. Low enough so that with her heart med, the Lanoxin, she was in danger of digitalis toxicity? What were the signs again? Six forty-five already, would she have time to get her textbook out of her locker? Sweat trickled between her shoulder blades, even though the regular staff nurses wore sweaters. Well, she had a minute to find out more about Zandra Loom. She flipped quickly to the social history page.

A widow. Mmmm, a good address. An address that went with the educated voice. Republican national committee woman in 1955. Donated to the west wing of the hospital. Republican, of course. She, Calla, could accept life's blows philosophically, if she'd been rich all her life like Mrs. Loom. She'd rather be a philanthropist any day than a nurse. A philanthropist in a halo cast? Yes—even so. Nursing puts you in danger.

Maybe she was the only one who thought so. Calla took note of the way the nurses talked to the patients, flip and easy, joking. Too familiar, her mother would have said. It was taking care of her mother that last year that gave her the idea, gave her elderly aunts the idea, that she ought to go into nursing. "You're so calm, and you have a kind smile," they all repeated, as if it were settled.

Go away, Aunt Elana said, Calla's mother needs her, then she closed the door in Darby's face, but there he still was, standing so close to the window he fogged it, his hand making a cut across his neck to take away the door slam. Aunt Elana, showing her yellow teeth in triumph, didn't see, but Calla did.

She hustled into 618 with her small tray of meds in fluted paper cups. Temperatures normal, same for pulse, respiration, and blood pressures. Calla loved the word 'normal,' which the day proved to be. Still, she went home so tired that her legs throbbed. After unplugging the phone, she collapsed on the couch and dropped off for at least fifteen minutes before she sat bolt upright and remembered that she'd forgotten to record the I and O, Input and Output, on Loom. Important enough to call about? Everything seemed important, so she left a message for the p.m. nurse and the station clerk, sounding impatient and amused said, "Okay, I'll tell her."

Calla lay back down and was just feeling vague and floaty again when the phone rang. Darby at a bar, saying how he loved her and hated her at the same time. She had no time for his Irish maudlin shit and unplugged the phone again. After a few minutes she sat up. If he couldn't talk to her, he'd get mad and come to the apartment. Enough to drink and he wouldn't give a damn about the restraining order. No sleep for her. Then she was sure to make another mistake, and would have to go through the longest two weeks of her life again in a year—another lifetime away. There was a Budget Motel across from the library.

As she stepped into the room, she thought, all mine. She got into the bathtub and ran the water as hot and high as she could stand, so only her face and the tips of her breasts and the soft mound of her stomach were out of water. It took her an hour to finish her bath, then she dressed in jeans and a sweatshirt and went out for dinner at Denny's, the one she used to go to with her friends from the library, which seemed a very long time ago. When she left, they'd presented her with a nurse doll holding a threatening syringe.

As she got into bed, she remembered—no alarm clock! She'd have to depend on the desk. "I must have a call at five!" She woke on her own at 5:30 a.m., drugged with sleep, but she dressed in five minutes, the toes of her supp hose still damp.

When she arrived at the hospital something nagged at the back of her head, something she'd forgotten, something much worse than forgetting the I and O, but she made herself get a roast beef sandwich and black coffee.

Though room 618 was not officially hers before report, she checked on them. "Can I do something for you, Mrs. Loom?" The elderly woman's face looked minutely askew in the wire geometry of her halo cast, her eyes very wide, and then, as before, heavy lidded.

"You're back. I wondered all this time why you left and didn't say goodbye."

"I told you goodbye yesterday. Perhaps it didn't register—you were very drowsy."

"When you died, you didn't say goodbye."

"It's me, Mrs. Loom, it's Calla."

"Calla. The nursing student. I've been talking nonsense. I didn't sleep well."

"She threw up last night." The roommate reached for a quilted bed jacket. "I took care of her. She told me not to get the nurse, but I would have if she'd gotten sick again."

"They don't have to know everything," Mrs. Loom said, "a shred of privacy, please."

Calla felt the same way about herself, but it was her job to pry, and yesterday she'd neglected to ask important questions.

A knock and "Calla?" It was the instructor. "They started report without you."

"I'm sorry!" Calla let go of Mrs. Loom's hands.

In the hall, Calla, wanting to bolt in two directions at once, said, "my patient was telling me something important. I should go back. I could take report from the staff nurse?"

"And waste her limited time? Hurry, catch it now."

Report on 618 was routine. No mention of nausea. "Excuse me," Calla said, and the team leader stopped the tape. "Mrs. Loom's roommate said Loom was sick, uh, had an emesis."

Outside the conference room, Calla caught up with Sue. "Mrs. Loom was so disoriented when she woke that she thought I was her dead daughter."

"Keep an eye out for her doctor. Good work, Calla, smile. You're doing fine."

"Thanks, Sue. I appreciate your support." Calla's eyes filled and she turned away. Being late wasn't serious, so why this nagging feeling? Possible *dig* toxicity! Her fingers damp, Calla paged through the drug book. Nausea! Disorientation!

Her heart beating in her throat, Calla slid the bell of her stethoscope under Mrs. Loom's left breast. Her apical pulse, her heart beat, was only 50.

"Calla, do you feel okay?" Sue asked, "You're white as a sheet."

"I'm holding the Lanoxin on Loom. I think she might have digitalis toxicity."

"What was her potassium when it came up yesterday?"

"It was low but not very. I don't remember exactly."

"Oh boy, I wish you'd . . . never mind. I'm just glad you caught this."

The chart was there for all to read—two shifts of nurses, Mrs. L's doctor, but Calla felt she was the weak link. She reported to the resident, who looked bored and ordered various blood tests and an electrocardiogram.

Somehow Calla got through the day and it was almost two thirty— only a final half hour to go and she would pass—but Sue was talking to the instructor. Calla felt her stomach knot. Sue was saying she hadn't reported the low potassium yesterday. The third strike. She kept on walking toward them. Better to get it over with.

"Calla!" Sue couldn't maintain her smile. "I've just been telling your instructor what a great job you do, how you picked up on the possible digitalis toxicity."

"You have great potential, Calla, but there's something I have to talk to you about." The instructor turned and led Calla into the chart room.

"I was checking the medications record, and I noticed that you didn't record Mrs. Loom's twelve o'clock Tagamet. Did you forget to give it?"

"No, I'm absolutely sure I gave it because I had three to give her and I checked them off on my assignment sheet as I gave them. Then I went to record them on the med record and I must have overlooked putting my initials in that particular box."

"What if Sue had looked at the meds record when you were at lunch and thought that you had not given it and gave it? That's not so terrible with this anti-ulcer med, but what if it had been a heart med?"

"Yes," Calla said, "that's bad." At last it was over. She felt lighter in her center. Now she had all the time in the world. "Am I out?"

"I'm sorry, Calla, yes. But I don't want this to discourage you. You'll be just fine as a nurse." The instructor's large pale eyes looked pensive. "If only you could relax."

While she waited for the instructor to return with the necessary paperwork, Calla reported off to Sue, who said, "I tried to make her change her mind." A hand on Calla's shoulder. "Don't let this get you down."

Calla finished her charting, and the words just flowed—medical abbreviations came from her pen as if she were a twenty-five year veteran.

The instructor gave Calla a written report of events. "Do you think that's fair?"

"Yes," Calla said. The instructor had praised her observational skills and her patient communication and rapport. "This is fair, but I'm confused about the way things work in nursing."

"Please go on."

"There was something else I failed to do, something that might have had far more serious consequences than failing to record a med. I should have brought the low potassium to Sue's attention and checked for the signs of dig toxicity a day before I did."

The instructor looked at her without quite making eye contact. "If you hadn't made your third mistake, would you have told me this?"

"I don't know," Calla said, then, "Of course not! Not unless my doing so would correct something seriously wrong with my patient!" Calla could picture herself slapping the instructor's smooth pink cheek. Didn't the woman have any idea of anything?

The instructor shook her head. "It's all a part of nursing ethics, Calla."

Calla went to tell 618 good-bye. "Mrs. Loom, let me turn you slightly to the other side. You've got to stay off your tailbone as much as possible." She wedged a pillow at her back, another between her knees. "Don't forget to do your bed exercises."

"No, I won't forget." Mrs. Loom smiled. "When I get out of this cast, I don't suppose I'll be seeing you at the library any more."

"No." Calla's mouth felt very dry. "I made a mistake today. It wasn't serious—I forgot to chart something, but now I have to wait to take my final clinical again, and I guess the best thing to do is get a job as a nursing assistant."

"Yes. You mustn't quit. I think you make a good nurse, much better than you were as a library aide. When I checked out my books, you were always staring into space. Maybe that's why you didn't remember me."

"Oh, but I did," Calla said, "but for some reason, I didn't think I ought to . . ."

"Remind us both of better days? I wonder. You, in any case—you look alert now."

The window behind her darkened as the snow came down. Calla thought she saw the double silver hoops of the halo cast turn, black then silver, spinning in the opaque light.

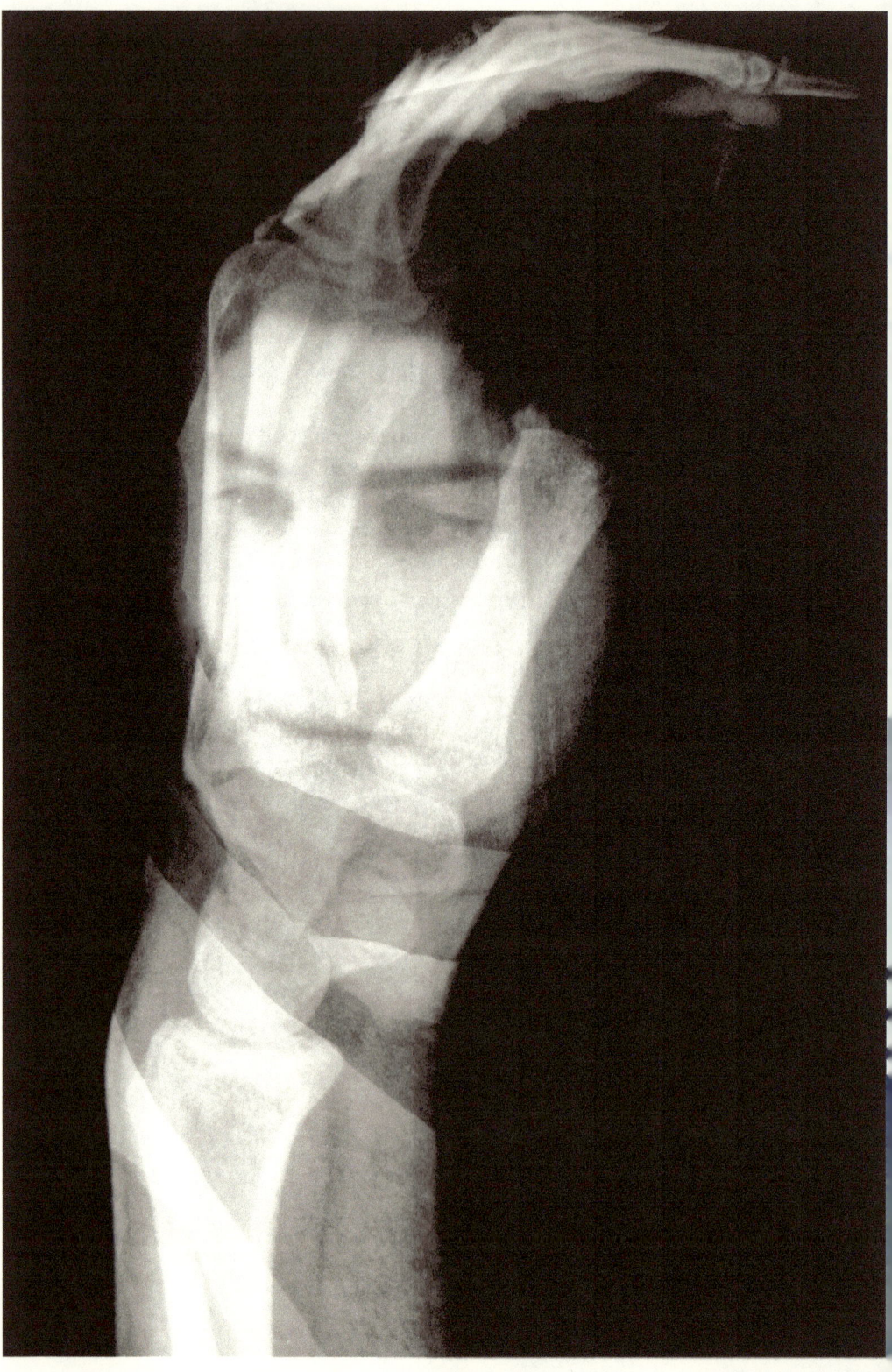

PHYLLIS A. LANGTON

COMPASSIONATE LISTENER

In the mid-1950s, I met Billy while working as a pediatric nurse in a university teaching hospital in southern California. There we received the most seriously ill children from the major west coast area and surrounding inland states. Billy, diagnosed with leukemia and lymphoma, a death sentence for children, was typical of our patients who had a variety of serious life-threatening diseases and conditions. Our patients needed special care, as did their families; many had traveled long distances with their children, hoping for miracles.

Medium height for his pre-teenager years, Billy was a sliver of a child. He had red hair, and soft, green eyes like a puppy. High cheekbones emphasized his long gaunt face, and a little-kid smile curled up the corner of his lips. Perhaps because of his father's notoriety as a comedian, Billy was not as out-going as some of the children, but he knew what was happening with the other kids on the ward, a frenzied place.

Herds of medical types made their daily rounds filling the four long hallways for hours at a time: attending physicians, special consultant physicians, accompanied by the usual flotilla of residents and interns. The level of teaching activity was exhilarating, yet exhausting with some people talking in medical language and waving their arms as they answered questions asked by the physicians. Others carried patient charts and wrote down orders given by the physician in charge.

And last, but not least, there were parents and sick children, some of whom were mobile. They liked to visit friends in their rooms, even though they were encouraged to remain in their own rooms. Of course, the phones rang constantly—a whirling dervish pace.

Because I was in my early twenties and open-natured, the children wanted to hug me when I arrived on the ward. I permitted this even though it was against ward policy. There were times when they needed to give and receive a human touch, their way of saying "Hello," and "I'm so happy to see you."

Billy had a unique way of getting my attention. As I walked briskly down the hall to get my work done, he shuffled up behind me in his noisy floppy slippers and playfully grabbed me from behind, his arms around my skinny waist. He held me until I stopped. We were a funny looking pair—two skinny broomsticks jammed together.

This game startled me at first, as he rubbed his skinny face into my bony back, breathing deep sighs, and sounding like a cat purring. I imagined he closed his eyes when he did this, and his soul felt great comfort. Maybe this was the way he greeted his family.

After he had been hanging on for a few seconds, I reached one hand around and tickled him until he let me go. "Hey, Billy. What's happening?" I asked.

He loved this ritual, and giggled loudly. "Gottcha!" he answered. "My father's coming today, and he's bringing lots of good stuff for everyone."

"Great. Do you want to have your friends in your room when he comes so you can have fun together?" I asked.

"Can we do that?" His face brightened.

"I think so if we don't interfere with the doctors' rounds," I said. "Let me check the schedule and see if you find out when your father plans to come."

One of the ward customs was to invite celebrities to entertain the children. During the 1950s, television became a popular pastime for children, including such shows as *Howdy Doody, Lassie, My Friend Flicka,* classic Disney cartons and the *Mickey Mouse Club.* The children often asked for the Mickey Mouseteers because they would bring big ears for the children to wear and keep. When the visits were arranged, I put as many children as possible in one big room, some in beds and chairs.

Billy's father was a big man on many dimensions. He was tall with a thick frame and ruddy complexion; his large eyes and bushy eyebrows floated above a smile as big as the face on the moon. Flat feet that never ended, with arms like an octopus, he reached out to touch the children when he did his tricks.

One of his favorite tricks was to use a huge air gun to blow my nurses' hat off my head. When he was successful, the game was to see who could catch the hat. The children whooped when my hat flew in different directions. He put the hat on the child who caught it, and then blew it off again, causing even more merriment among the kids.

But a real challenge for me was when he tried to blow my heavy, starched skirt up from my legs. I ran around the crowded room while he chased me with this air gun.

"Stop! Stop!" I hollered, while the children squealed and jumped up and down in their beds. Not only was the air cold on my legs, it blew everything on the floor into circles, including the children's slippers, and anything dropped on the floor. Spirits were high. For a time, the children forgot they were in the hospital.

Billy stood in the background as the other children enjoyed their time with his father. But he always tried to protect me from the air gun by running in front of me. I could only imagine how exciting and high-spirited life must have been for Billy living with such a lively comedian.

His father also brought boxes of comic books, coloring books with crayons and small paperbacks to read. Some of the children called him Santa Claus because he brought multiple bags of presents.

Twice he brought treats from his trip to Hawaii. "Here, here," he teased me in his comic, clown voice. "Open, open the can." He knew I didn't like what was in the can.

"Yucky, yucky. Barbequed sparrows in a can!" As I said this he started to open the can so I could see them. I ran to the other side of the room. "That is terrible! Get those birds out of here!" The children laughed even though they didn't know why they were laughing, as they caught on to the apparent teasing between us.

The children hollered when Billy's father pretended to take off my nose and put it behind my ear. I said, "Oh, no, don't take my nose. I need it! Put it back!" The children yelled, "Give her back her nose!" He pretended to put it back and then he started another game to get them laughing.

Then he gave them bags of popcorn, and the munching began.

One afternoon when I arrived, Billy was waiting for me. He grabbed my waist as usual, but this time he wouldn't let go when I tickled him. His kneading grip was different from his playful grip, and suggested he was reflecting some inner hurt. I had no idea what had occurred to put him in this state.

When he finally let go and I saw the tears in his eyes, I took his hand and led him up the hallway to a quieter area. There, we could sit and talk at a small table with two little chairs. Billy seemed unusually fragile; the helplessness of his eyes pierced my soul. "Sit here, Billy, and I will get us a soda."

I helped him into the chair, hurried to the kitchen, and told my co-worker where I would be in case I was needed for an emergency.

When I returned, Billy jumped into my lap, stuttering as his story burst out. His friend, Larry, had died that morning. "The nurses put us in a room and wouldn't tell us why. They pulled the curtains, closed the doors, and ran down the hall with him on a stretcher," he said. "We peeked through the curtains, but we never had a chance to tell him goodbye. Why wouldn't they let us tell him goodbye? We need to wave goodbye to our friends when they leave."

I realized what he was telling me. This ritual of hiding the death, or of seeing a stretcher with the body racing by made death a bigger mystery. This really scared him and the other children.

I held him close because I could see the tightness in his face; his huge eyes were fixed in a stare. The tenderness he aroused in me was overwhelming. I also saw that his physical condition had deteriorated markedly in the last three days. He was more fragile, had lost weight, and deeper creases showed on his chalk-white face. The body odor that escaped from his open bathrobe was rancid. His limbs felt cold, and his balance was unsteady. I wondered if his reaction to the death of his friend and how it had been handled was exacerbated by his physical changes.

He was shaking when he said, "Will this happen to me? Will I die here and ride down the hall on a stretcher? I'm scared."

"I'm sorry about Larry and that you didn't get to tell him goodbye, Billy. What can I do to help you feel better?"

"I want to go home and see my friends," he said.

"When? Let me check with the head nurse and have her call your doctor and your father, if that's okay with you. Perhaps there's a way you can come back in for your lab tests every other day or so. Do you want me to do that?" Seeing the change in his condition and feeling his fragile body, I felt he needed to be home with his family to share the precious time remaining in his life.

"Yes, now," he whispered.

When I lifted him off my lap, he looked like he would collapse. I took him back to his room, tucked him into bed, and rubbed his back so he would take a short nap. Moist-eyed, I told him I would be back as soon as I could.

After listening to me plead Billy's case, including his fear of dying that night, his fear of being run down the hall dead on a stretcher, and the physical signs of his failing condition, the head nurse called his doctor and family who made the decision for him to leave the hospital around 8 p.m.

Later, when I returned to tell Billy, he hadn't touched his dinner. He was sitting on his bed with his legs dangling over the side. His shoulders sagged with his burden, his eyes stared at the floor, and his shriveled body nearly disappeared into his bathrobe. When he looked up and saw my big smile, he knew the news was good. He grabbed my waist, this time from the front, and held on. As the lost and solemn expression disappeared, the rosy color returned to his face. He was going home.

After Billy left with his father, I grabbed my sandwich from the refrigerator, a cup of coffee, and hurried down to the nurses' lounge for a late dinner break, and to review for my exam the next day. But the experience with Billy haunted me. I feared I would never see him again. I needed to sort out what had awakened in me during the weeks I had cared for him.

I gulped down my coffee and sandwich. Rather than writing my usual clinical nursing notes—I would write them later—I began to write my reflections of this powerful experience.

Thinking back on my childhood, I remembered being shuttled from birth in 1933 to foster homes during the Great Depression. Then I was sent to a children's home, and in 1946 out into the world at age thirteen. I didn't learn the value of the human touch as a means to connect and communicate with others. Nobody patted me on the head affectionately as a child; nobody told me I was cute. Nobody hugged me or put their arms around me when I hurt. I had no laps to sit on.

When Billy trusted me by sharing his deep grief about the death of his friend and how the nurses handled that death, I knew I couldn't fix the whole problem, but I could fix a small part of it by pleading his case to go home that evening. Billy showed me how important it is to be both competent and caring. Then you are able to do the best for your patients. He showed me that sometimes there is a need for human touch. It is a way of connecting so that immediate pain, loneliness, or fear can be reduced. He showed me that fear can do terrible things to people—especially to vulnerable people. He was terrified he would die and be rushed down the hall on a stretcher, without his friends knowing what had happened to him.

I vowed that in the future, when I first met my patients, I would begin by listening to them tell me their needs—and the fears that surface when people are hospitalized and in some cases, dying.

Billy didn't realize he had given me one of the greatest gifts of my life: a change in myself. He changed how I would practice from then on.

Two days after he left the hospital, Billy's father called to ask if Billy's favorite nurses could care for him at his home. His condition was grave. Unfortunately, I was near the end of final exams, but I promised to be there in two days. Billy died at home before I was able to be there to care for him. While I felt devastated for his family, I felt a moment of peace because he died at home with his family.

CLAUDETTE MORK SIGG

THE DARKNESS IN SISTER MERCY

Her cap crowned her head, a wedding cake confection—
or, perhaps, a battleship sailing into intentional catastrophe.
White hands crisped down her uniform, skirt and all. Nothing
clung to her, not a thread or speck of dirt.

Cool blue eyes identified, registered, filed away
each small patient in the children's ward,
a tumor here, a blood clot there, a broken leg,
leukemia and tonsils, cancer eating up a small brain.

She cruised past those who would live,
harbored herself by the bedsides of the dying, feeding
on them with her smiles, her little jokes, the pat
of her hand, the consolation of teddy bears.

She took away plastic containers of chicken soup,
applesauce, whispered to them, "You don't want this
anymore, do you?" No one else heard her say, what's left
will go in the garbage, and that will be the end of it.

NINA GABY

THE INVENTORIES WE KEEP

The alcohol van would drop the gurney off at the ED entrance, throw some paperwork at the security guard and take off. We'd recognize Joseph by his bare feet sticking out from under the sheet, gray and scaly, always worrying that we'd lift the sheet up and he wouldn't be breathing. Triage never sent him over for medical clearance, just the fast track to Psych, and we never questioned it. Every place has its rituals. It was just Joseph. I had never heard the term "frequent flyer" until I was asked to come work down in the Psych ED when I was in grad school. Joseph made our Top Ten. We would worry when we hadn't seen him in a while. When he was around there'd be the betting between the nurses and doctors and techs as to what his BAL would be this time. I won once with a 438, an old street address.

"You know he's going to be dead one of these days," Nancy my hardcore psych nurse colleague would say. And then one of the residents would tell the story of the guy with the 700 and we'd order pizza. It rarely varied, our rituals on a Saturday night.

We all move along, each in our way, wondering what kind of job we are doing but little time for narcissistic meandering in a busy city hospital. Lucky if you have a good supervisor who doesn't use your vulnerabilities as a teachable moment for the rest of the staff, or if you have a couple of like-minded colleagues you can place bets or share a Kleenex with.

I was not particularly special to Joseph's care. Thiamine, Haldol, Ativan, socks and a sandwich. Basic nursey stuff. I took it in stride that there was no help for him. Joseph would die, be found some spring under a melting pile of snow. Those tough images were fine. It was a busy city hospital. Not like TV although I was new at this and pretended it to be. And Joseph was never a therapy patient or a member of one of my treatment groups. Just someone I found socks for and told what his blood alcohol level was each time, mentioned his liver and his brain, and asked him if he wanted a referral.

Which he always did but never followed up on.

It was somewhat unfortunate that at a very young age I'd watched a movie on our little black and white television set about people looking for a place called Shangri-La. Until adulthood I really thought it was an actual place. No matter that people shriveled up into dust as payment for finding it. The idea stuck in my head that if one climbed high enough there would be something there. Epiphanies, rewards. Certain expectations were laid down. But there were years of Joseph, years of crisis patients, the same stories over and over again. The twenty year old with lupus and absolutely no one in the world willing to watch her three toddlers, so we had to do her therapy sessions around their sticky outstretched hands and then she would lug the strollers back up the bus steps. The black grandmas that were so ashamed about being angry that they wanted to kill themselves, church be damned. Because after bringing up their own kids who they would always lose to crack, they were now saddled with their grandkids. When all they wanted to do was get their Nursing Assistant certificates but now they had "sugar" and "blood pressure" and crack babies to care for. There were people whose kids choked to death on birthday balloons while the adults were getting drunk. There were first breaks. Second breaks. Thwarted brilliance.

One gets used to these things. Even the life changing moments aren't that pivotal in the scheme of these things. You don't even realize that you've had a moment. The moment is usually stolen because of all the other things you have to be doing. Pleading pre-authorization. CYA documentation. The moment may come later when you tell your spouse about your day or you bring it to supervision, just glad you've got something good to talk about. You travel along simultaneous planes, you lose yourself in the self-assessment process, filing it somewhere.

But then over the years maybe it becomes bigger. Twenty years later you find yourself telling the story to someone you are supervising. Or as you sit with hopelessness your mind crawls around. You think of the moment that didn't make it all worth it, let's be honest, the paycheck is supposed to do that, but has become part of the bedrock of your own professional mythology.

Joseph reappeared once again to make my own Top Ten, that inventory we don't even realize we keep. After not seeing him for several years, having moved on to an office a quarter of a mile down the hall from the Psych ED, and having assumed of course that he had been found under thawing gravel,

I didn't think about Joseph any more. Life was tough, there were DRGs and turf struggles and a difficult pregnancy. Stupid administrative decisions. Never enough time to make a difference. Crack. Refractory symptoms. Revolving doors. A little strange bleeding.

I stood outside my office one day, an office with a window, knowing that as soon as I left on maternity leave I would lose the window and come back to mean uncertainty. It was mid-afternoon and I couldn't have any more caffeine. I was lost in my own miserable thoughts.

I felt a tap on my shoulder, turned around to see a black man with stylish eyeglasses, really nice shoes, in a three-piece suit, smiling at me. "I'm sorry, do I know you?" I asked, a reflexively protective hand to my stomach. He continued to smile. "I'm really sorry but I don't know who you are." It was outpatient Psych so it could have been anybody, it could have been possibly a danger, I suppose, someone standing so close, smiling so hard.

"I've been waiting for this moment for two years" the familiar voice said. "I've been waiting two years for you not to recognize me." It was Joseph, of course.

He spent a few moments telling me about his recovery, his job in a community action non-profit, and then politely said that he would let me get back to work. He thanked me, I, of course, thanked him harder.

It was a big moment, but not big enough to keep me in health care for more than a few more years. After a while we moved to Vermont, bought an old country inn, a cliché that didn't work out. So the real life changing moment came when I had to go back into health care to survive, messing around in those files in my head, counting off my Top Ten on my ten fingers to remind myself, okay, this is okay.

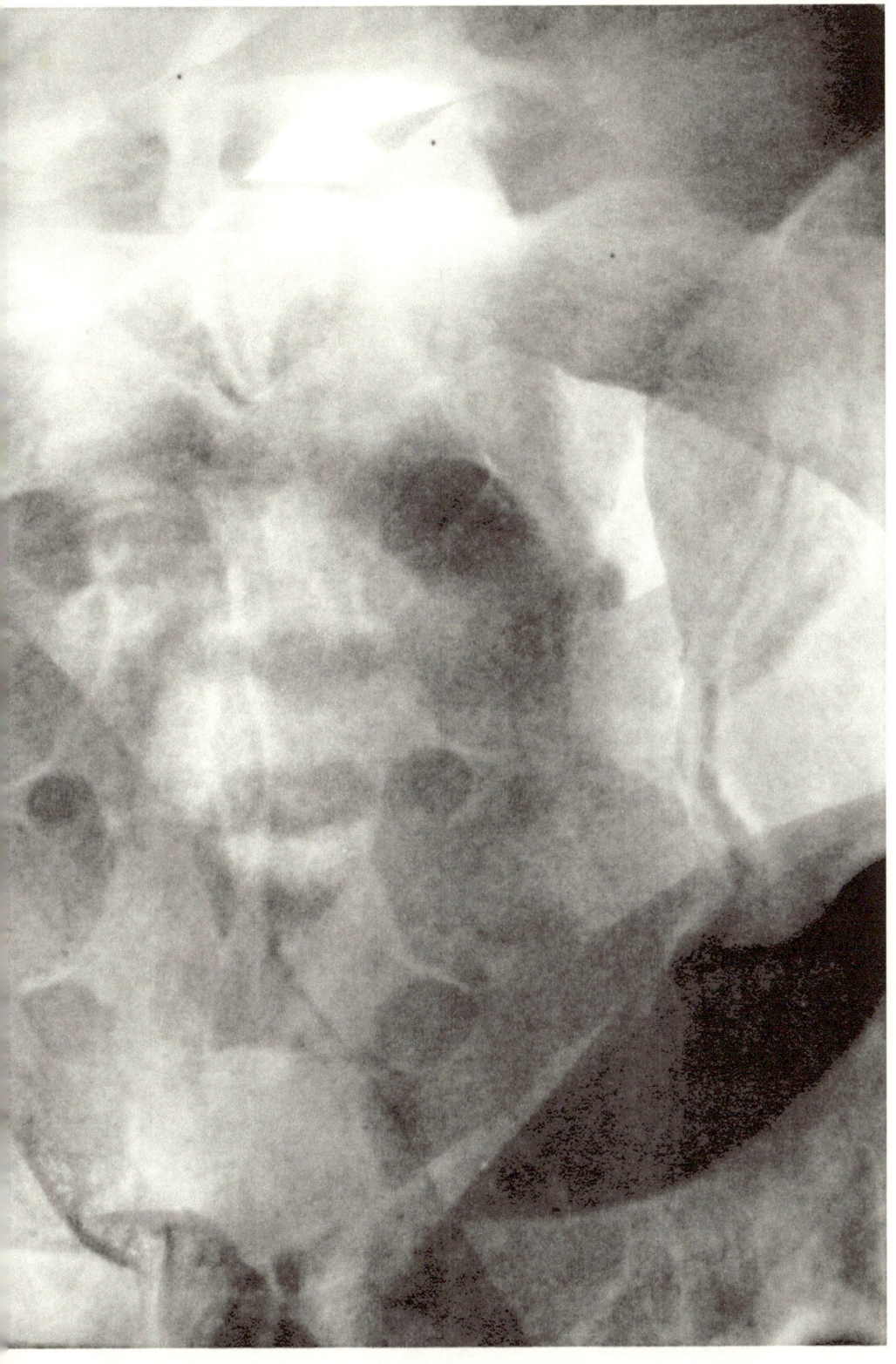

ROBERT J. KUS

RICH MURRAY, M.D.

After almost forty-four years as an R.N. in clinical and university settings, I have known many physicians. None, though, have made more of an impression on me than Rich Murray.

I first met Rich when he was dating my sister, Chris. He was establishing his practice in Internal Medicine in Green, Ohio, a suburb of Akron. I immediately liked him, for he was a down-to-earth type of guy with a great sense of humor. He thoroughly enjoyed life, and was very sensitive and focused.

After he got married, he and Chris began having children. In time, they joined a non-denominational church and became active members.

Each day, Rich would get up around 4 a.m. and, with a cup of coffee, read the Bible, reflect on what he read, and pray to the Lord.

Around 5:30 a.m., Rich would make rounds at the hospital to see if his patients needed anything. Afterwards, he usually took medical students to breakfast in the hospital cafeteria. Medical students, lowest on the medical totem pole, were often treated with distain by many of the medical staff. They loved Rich, though, because he was always kind to them. He listened to their stories, laughed at their jokes, and commiserated with their trials and tribulations. He never made fun of their questions; rather, he answered all questions with great respect to the students.

This quality of Rich was not reserved, though, to medical students. This apparently was a deeply ingrained part of his personality, for he treated all people like that, be they receptionists, nurses, janitors, clerks. Today there is a TV-radio personality named Clark Howard. Clark's voice and consistent kindness towards others mirrors Rich's approach to people in remarkable ways. Even their voices and the rhythm of their talk is the same.

Rich was also a strong champion of the underdogs of society, especially the poor and disenfranchised. Frequently he would mark "No charge" on patients' records when he suspected they were having a tough time financially.

Rich's priorities were very clear. He cherished his God, his family, and his profession—in that order.

One of the customs that Rich and Chris had was to take one of their children away on a weekend holiday by themselves. Sometimes Chris and Rich would do that together, and other times they would do that separately. On one occasion, Rich took his younger son on a trip to Myrtle Beach, SC. Though they had a good time, Rich began experiencing abdominal discomfort.

When Rich and his son got back to Ohio, Rich had a friend of his give him a physical to see what might be causing his "stomach upset." Within three days, his friend and other physicians diagnosed Rich with liver cancer. As it turned out, the part of the liver that was not cancerous was cirrhotic from a needle stick he had experienced as a medical student.

The downhill journey was rapid, and Rich spent his last days in the hospital where he worked. Ironically, the terminal care policies of the hospital that the staff followed had been developed by Rich and his committee.

To the end, Rich was cheerful and always concerned about the welfare of his family, staff, and friends.

Four weeks after being diagnosed with cancer, Rich died.

The funeral home visitation went for a few days. When I arrived, the funeral home people said that they had stopped counting how many people had come for visitation after the first two thousand people!

The ride to the cemetery was amazing as squads of police tried to keep the line of cars, winding their way as far as the eye could see, moving safe and sound.

Rich has been gone a few years now, and his four children have become incredible human beings. Rich touched the lives of so many people, and every once in a while, when I'm dealing with particularly difficult people as a parish priest, I ask myself, "What would Rich do?"

In reflecting on Rich's life, I do so through the prism of a psychiatric-mental health nurse, sociologist, professor, and Catholic priest.

As an R.N., I was always very impressed at Rich's kindness, sensitivity, and compassion towards his patients and towards staff. These qualities, which I associate with good nursing, are sometimes absent or minimal in physicians who may be arrogant and emotionally distant. Rich demonstrated every day how one can be a compassionate human being and physician at the same time; the two are not mutually exclusive.

As a sociologist, I was always impressed with how well he grasped his adult social roles and how he honored each of them to the best of his ability. Though he played many social roles in life—son, uncle, friend, committee member and chairperson—the social roles he cherished most were those of Christian, husband, father, and physician.

As an adult, everything he did flowed from his Christian faith. All his actions reflected the values of his belief system, values such as putting his family before his work, honesty, integrity, sensitivity, compassion, and fortitude.

I was impressed that he was able to have such a great balance in his roles of family man and private practice physician. Though he ran a successful private Internal Medicine practice, which requires an incredible amount of knowledge, time and dedication, he always had plenty of time to devote to his wife and children. Never did any one of his social roles suffer. This is in stark contrast to the workaholic stereotype of a father who works so hard making a living that he becomes a stranger to his family, and it is also in stark contrast to the worker who is so concerned with family matters that he or she is on the phone to family members throughout the day on company time.

As a priest, I was very impressed at Rich's leadership skills as head of the domestic church. The domestic church, or "first level" of church, is the family. In Catholic Christian theology, every person becomes part of the "priesthood of all believers" at his or her baptism when the Holy Spirit enters the person and brings an array of amazing gifts.

Most baptized persons grow up to start families, domestic churches. They are the priests of the church, and their children are the flock. Priests do many things in their role as priests. They, for example, are storytellers. They tell stories of Jesus and some of his adventures and parables. They talk about God and God's awesome creation. They tell stories of the saints and other heroes of the faith.

As priests, parents teach children basic values such as how to say "Please" and "Thank you," how to share toys with others, how not to hit each other in the head with blocks, and the like.

Priests teach their flock how to chat with God; this is called praying. Like other priests, Rich taught his children both formal prayers (those written in books such as the Lord's Prayer or Our Father), and spontaneous prayers.

By the time the children were two or three, they could lead the assembly (family) in spontaneous prayer around the dining room table.

Priests of the domestic church also teach their children the meaning of the symbols of their faith such as the meaning of the cross, and they teach them how to celebrate rituals of the faith such as the lighting of the candles on an Advent wreath.

Parents as priests also teach their children how to read the Bible and apply it to their daily lives. Rich and Chris did this most remarkably. Today all of Rich's children can turn to the Bible for guidance on any topic.

Finally, priests of the domestic church take their flock to the second level of church. Catholics call this their parish, and Protestants call it their local church. Rich and Chris took their children to a non-denominational mega church in Akron, Ohio called The Chapel.

In every respect, Rich was a terrific leader of the domestic church with his wife, Chris. As a result, they produced four beautiful children.

Finally, as a university professor, I was always impressed with Rich's gentleness and clarity in teaching. Harshness and ridicule were foreign to him. Rather, he taught medical students and his children with patience, respect, and kindness. As a result of this teaching style, his "pupils" learned and learned well.

There are so many people like Rich who live their lives hidden from the spotlight of fame and fortune. That's sad, for their lives are so very inspirational and illustrative. So many young parents would be able to learn so much from knowing about Rich's life and the lives of others like him. I, certainly, believe I'm a much richer person for encountering him on my own life journey. And for that, I am very grateful.

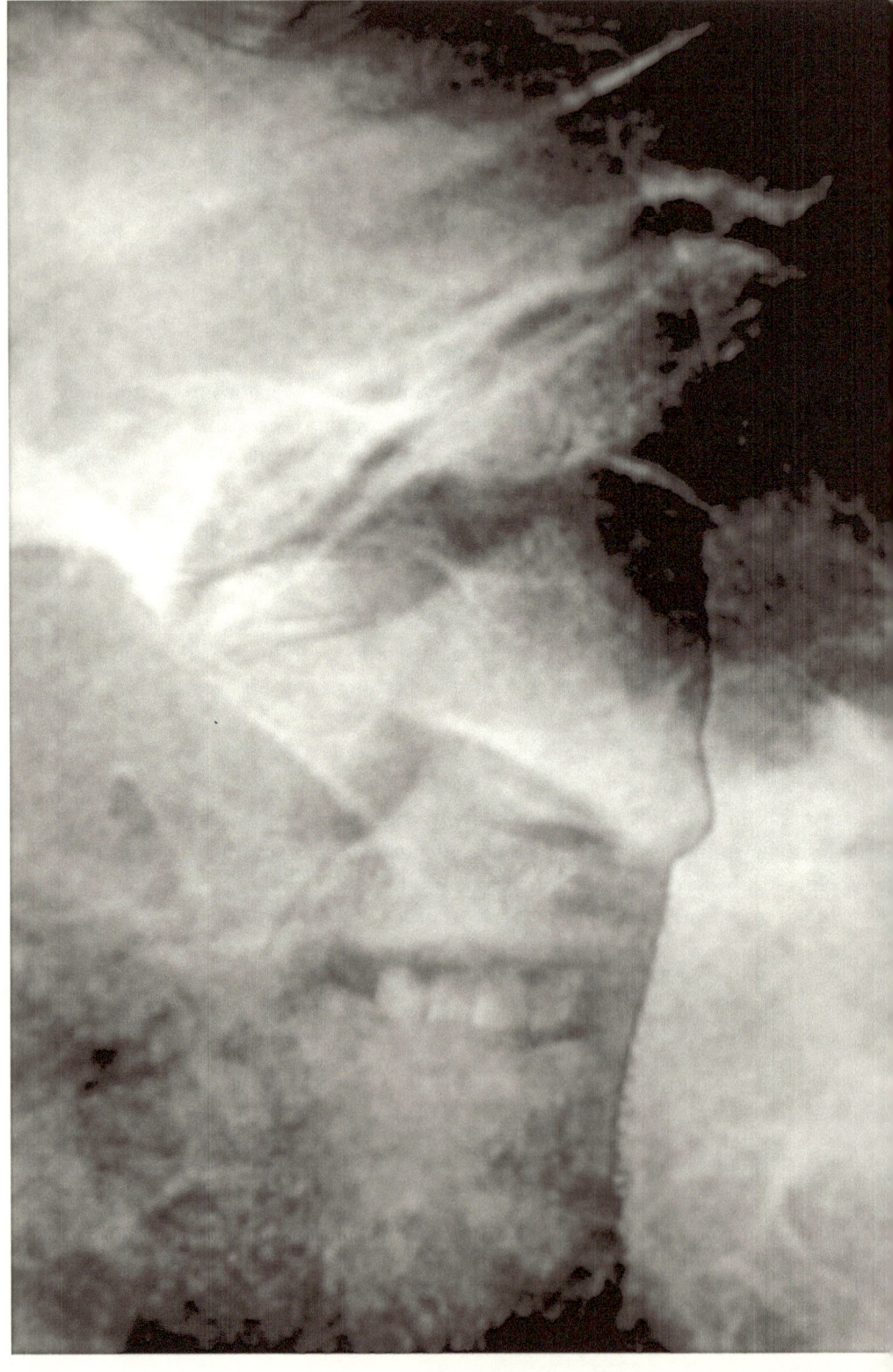

JOEL PECKHAM

CHRONIC

"That sounds like a death-sentence."

For a second I let Father Tom's comment linger in the air. It's not often that I am struck silent, if ever. And after all, I merely stated the obvious, what I've been saying for years—what every therapist and every friend and even the minister at the bedside in Mass General has said and says every day:

"I will live with it for the rest of my life."

Rachael and I are getting married and as Episcopalians we are going through required premarital counseling at Amelia's Church of the Good Samaritan on Olive Branch Rd. across from the pawn shop and the Karate Dojo in a small Cincinnati suburb dominated by Methodists, Baptists, and Catholics. We sit, holding hands in the tiny office in the back amid the muted blaring of impatient drivers who lurch forward only to be stopped again by another light, another car trying to turn against traffic, by some pedestrian scampering among the cars.

"Or a life-sentence—like something a judge would say to a criminal."

I like Father Tom. I like his white beard and his dramatic way. I like his theater doctorate and how he hugs me when he sees me—too tight, like an overly affectionate uncle, occasionally planting a kiss on my cheekbone. I like how he ends every service by crouching down at the back of the hall and winding up, a centerfielder throwing a ball toward the plate, before shouting, not like a priest but some God-crazed Appalachian evangelist, *hallelujah, Hallelujah. HA LLE LU JAH!* As my New England Unitarian progenitors laugh in the stony graves.

"Have you thought about giving it up?" he says, stroking his beard and leaning so far back in his swivel chair that I feel as if it might just tip over.

"Giving it to God."

"No," I want to say. But I nod. I smile. Tell him, "I'll think about it." I don't say, "I don't want God to have it. Its mine," like a little boy with a new ball, afraid to share. I'm not afraid to share. Anyone can play with my ball. But you see, it's my ball. Mine. I take it home with me. I get to carry it with me everywhere I go. Forever. God will have to go get someone else's. Or get His own. After all, there is plenty of grief and pain and suffering in the world—what with Tsunamis and Earthquakes in Iran, Hurricane Katrina, AIDs in Africa, Bird-Flu, and the war in Iraq. He doesn't need mine.

No.

We are talking about Cyrus and Susan again. About grief. My grief. But at this moment Father Tom reminds me not of a spiritual healer but of every medical doctor I have dealt with over the past four years.

"You know there's a new therapy."

"There's this drug I want you to try"

"What they do is insert this needle in your spine."

"There's a very small chance of side-effects—numbness, sexual dysfunction, but for many patients . . ."

"It's not a cure, but it should give you some relief."

"I can help you."

"Do you want to suffer forever—needlessly?"

"I can help you."

"Do you want to suffer?"

Neurontin. Percocet. Oxycodone. Serequel. Tramadol. Tylenol with Codeine.

I am a chronic pain sufferer. One of millions of Americans who live every day with discomfort that sends many of us folding into ourselves like nightflowers, or—like the drivers outside—lurching angrily from doctor to doctor, starting hopefully only to stop abruptly when the painkiller doesn't work, or it makes us sick or causes anxiety. When we find blood in our urine or can't sleep for a couple of days. And yes, there are a few—not many but some—some of us who simply take the last trip to the medicine cabinet and a final appointment with one of those attractive bottles of pills meant to make their lives bearable.

And I guess that I am a chronic grief sufferer too. Though in my own mind, physical and emotional pain are so much a part of the same fabric that I would not even try to unravel them.

In the first months after the accident—still bed-ridden with nothing to stop the brush fire in my right foot and nothing to halt the imagery of shattered windshields and fresh graves from flickering and flashing in the magic lantern of memory—I would imagine myself sunk deeply into the mattress as if I had landed there from some great height, a skydiver whose chute had failed to open, a shattered body impressed on a cool wet field.

In his great poem, "Falling," James Dickey imagines the last moments of a flight attendant who *"was swept through an emergency door that suddenly sprang open."* Her back broken, lying in moonlight in an open field she "Feels herself go   go toward   go outward   breathes at last fully / Not   and tries less   once   tries   tries   AH, GOD—"

How lucky, I would think, it would be to let go, to have flown like Cyrus off into the night sky. Was it like that for him that dark night in Jordan when our van hit the sand-truck? Flight. Impact. A last heroic becoming. I'd try to sink, to slip downward through the mattress. Be one with the earth with him. With Susan. But the needles in my foot would insist: "You're not going anywhere!" Scream: "alive—you will live." No death sentence for you. As if the poem had not ended at all, but was prelude. So the stewardess, back broken, organs mangled, mind warped by what she had seen on the way down, miraculously survived—forced to live with the constant reminder that we are not birds. Icarus' death was a blessing to Icarus. We do not have the story of his father's struggle to live with that death.

That was my story, or part of it.

Though I could sink no further, the hole I had formed in falling was deep, its walls sheer. Pain isolates. So does grief. The persistent nerve pain worried the doctors. And the trancelike quiet I retreated into worried my father who would look in from the bedroom door and order me up on crutches and out of the house. "You can't just lie there, damn it." One day he purchased a computer and placed it by my bed. "You're a writer. Now write." The blank screen would mock me for hours. He set up appointments with the pain clinic at Mass General and psychotherapy with a counselor who worked with him at the local high school. Self-help books rose in piles around the bed—*A Walk In the Woods, The Power of Now, A Case for Faith.*

In group therapy the father whose son committed suicide by leaping from his college dormitory wept and stammered. "He landed on his feet and everything was shattered from the hips down—like he was made of matchsticks." And he hammered his fist onto the table in front of him, the crash of skin and bone on wood reverberated off the stone walls of the church. Always, there was the implicit question, *What did I do wrong?* And the parents would nod their heads in support, bonded in their effort to understand the loss of their children. And they would stare at the crosses on the walls, their eyes imploring *Why us, God?* I nodded with them, saying nothing. I was with them but not of them. Distanced not only by circumstance—*not just a son, a son and a wife*—or by perspective—*I know what I did wrong*—but by the medical haze of oxycodone—*I am here and not here.* Sometimes I would sit in the circle and imagine myself floating around the room, slipping down in to the floorboards like water, or disappearing all at once into a thousand pieces, an airy vapor. Abracadabra. Hocus Pocus. Then the nerves would fire—dragging me back. *You are here. You are right here.*

At the pain center doctors would show me what was going on in my body, using plastic models: "When your femeral head broke through the acetabular socket, shattering the pelvis, part of that displaced bone crushed the sciatic nerve." *I know this already.* "This resulted in peripheral neuropathy, a spontaneous firing of the peripheral nerves—that's what's causing the burning sensation." *No shit.* "The good thing in your case is that the pain is limited to your foot." *I want to laugh.* "And you're taking it remarkably well. You don't seem afraid. You're not catastrophizing like some people." *I want to laugh.* "We've seen much worse." *I want to laugh.*

In the lobby, as I filled out the pain chart, circling the faces that most matched my own—from smiling and yellow to frowning and red—a woman who could have been anywhere from twenty-five to fifty folded like a lawn chair and hugged her knees to her chest, crumpling her chart into a ball. Her face glistened with sweat and, though dressed well, she smelled as if she had been sleeping in the street. "I just can't stand it anymore," she said over and over again. "I just came in for a hip replacement and now everything hurts. I'm afraid to move. And the damned doctors. They tell me nothing's wrong with me. Like its all in my head." I listened, saying nothing, watching the desperation in her eyes, glancing from my chart to her face, trying to make a match. "So what's wrong with you?"

On the drive home my mother and I went over the possible treatment options detailed in glossy pamphlets that reminded me of travel brochures to exotic destinations. And in some ways they were just that, each one promising relief and rest. Each one saying, "I can help you." My mother was terrified by my suffering. Terrified by the doctors who'd tell us, "you might always have some pain, maybe a great deal." Terrified by the way my cheeks turned ashen, by my weight-loss, by the long hours lying in bed, staring at ceiling, by the way I answer her hopeful question "are you OK honey?" with a blank stare, the calm and honest answer: "I may never be OK again. And you need to stop waiting for me be OK." I'm not trying to hurt her. But her hope seems like an expectation that I cannot satisfy. I can't pull off the lie. I can't look her in the eyes and say, "Yes Mom, I'm fine." Or "Don't worry, I'll be alright." I don't know if I will ever be fine. I'm tired of false hope. I'm tired of lies.

"What about the spinal injection?" she asked brightly, looking forward over the cars in front of her, glancing from the windshield to the rearview to me, then glancing back to me, weaving through the busy traffic on 93 South. I wanted to tell her how beautiful and brave I found her in that moment. I wanted to kiss her on the cheek and thank her.

Then I wanted to jump out of the window of the car and fall into the bay beneath us.

"No."

"What do you mean, 'No'? Won't you just consider it? The doctor said . . . "

"I'm not going back there. I'm not putting a needle in my spine so they can inject God knows what into me. Didn't you listen to the side-effects?"

"*Possible* side-effects. Why can't you be more optimistic. Do you want to suffer forever? I can't think of you in pain, Jo."

I wish I could have told her then the hard truth. That suffering is not a curse or some terrible burden, but a condition of life. It is life as is Joy and Pleasure. We can accept that without cynicism. As I watched my mother navigate the angry congested artery leading out of the city I thought of all that seething, writhing, life—the many lives desperate for movement, and climbing over each other to one destination or another. All of it heading forward in a rush—to nowhere perhaps, but somewhere, and together with us among them.

The hundred-thousand pins stabbing and slicing my feet, the glass-shard insects crawling up my legs kept stabbing, "now," slicing, "now," crying "now." They would not be denied or ignored. There was no past. No future for them. No moment far off in some distant country where and when the pain would stop except in death.

The acceptance of pain was my first tentative step on the crushed bottle path ahead of me. I knew this to be true. That to search for an end to pain would be endless—one drug after another, one hospital room after another. I stared at my mother. She seemed so frightened. So frantic and desperate. I felt badly for her, responsible to her, and to my father and every kind pair of searching eyes that only wanted to see me stop hurting, but for the first time in a long while I felt strong. *I can deal with this.* To accept is not to hold on, but to embrace, to embrace one's condition. It was also to embrace a new identity.

I am a chronic sufferer. One of twenty million with my specific condition. And this translated to another acceptance. I am a widower and a man who lost a child. And another: I am a father still. I am a man. I am not one of twenty million, but one of a hundred millions. Sitting in that car sealed off from a rainy, cold, New England April, I stared at the road in front of us, clogged and clotted with obstacles, and so many people going over them every day, each with his or her own burden to carry with them. I was one of them and the road was right in front of us, right there. I was anxious to travel it.

I stopped going to the group therapy sessions as well and while I still continued my meetings with my counselor, they began to take on a different aspect. Conversation became less about rehashing the past than about managing the future—how and where I would work. How I would take care of my son. Each day was rife with dragons to slay—real and imagined.

There would be mornings, many mornings when getting out of bed would seem as impossible as flight, but I would swing my sore hip over the edge of the mattress and lower my feet into the acid bath of the floor, manipulate the sock aid and the grabber and maneuver my pants over my feet, pull them up, then reach for my pants, stand and make my way out.

There would be hours in bed, when the entire world was reduced to a spot on the ceiling as I tried to lift my foot two inches, then three inches, four.

There would be setbacks, hard falls down stairs, wood floors, on ice.

But I would keep standing and rising.

To mornings when my son, waking, groggy from sleep would crawl into bed with me, burrowing into me, saying "Daddy, guess what?"

"What honey?"

"Guess."

"You love me?"

"Yes," and giggle and snuggle harder, too hard to the point of pain and I would love it.

There would be love and the making of love.

And it would all bring me here, with Rachael, to talk about marriage and the future, my foot shouting, "now," the world around me, crying "now, now, now."

"Think about it," Father Tom says, wisely, leaning back. Pulling on his beard.

"I will live with it for the *rest of my life.*"

"I will *live* with it for the rest of my life."

"I will *live with it* . . . . "

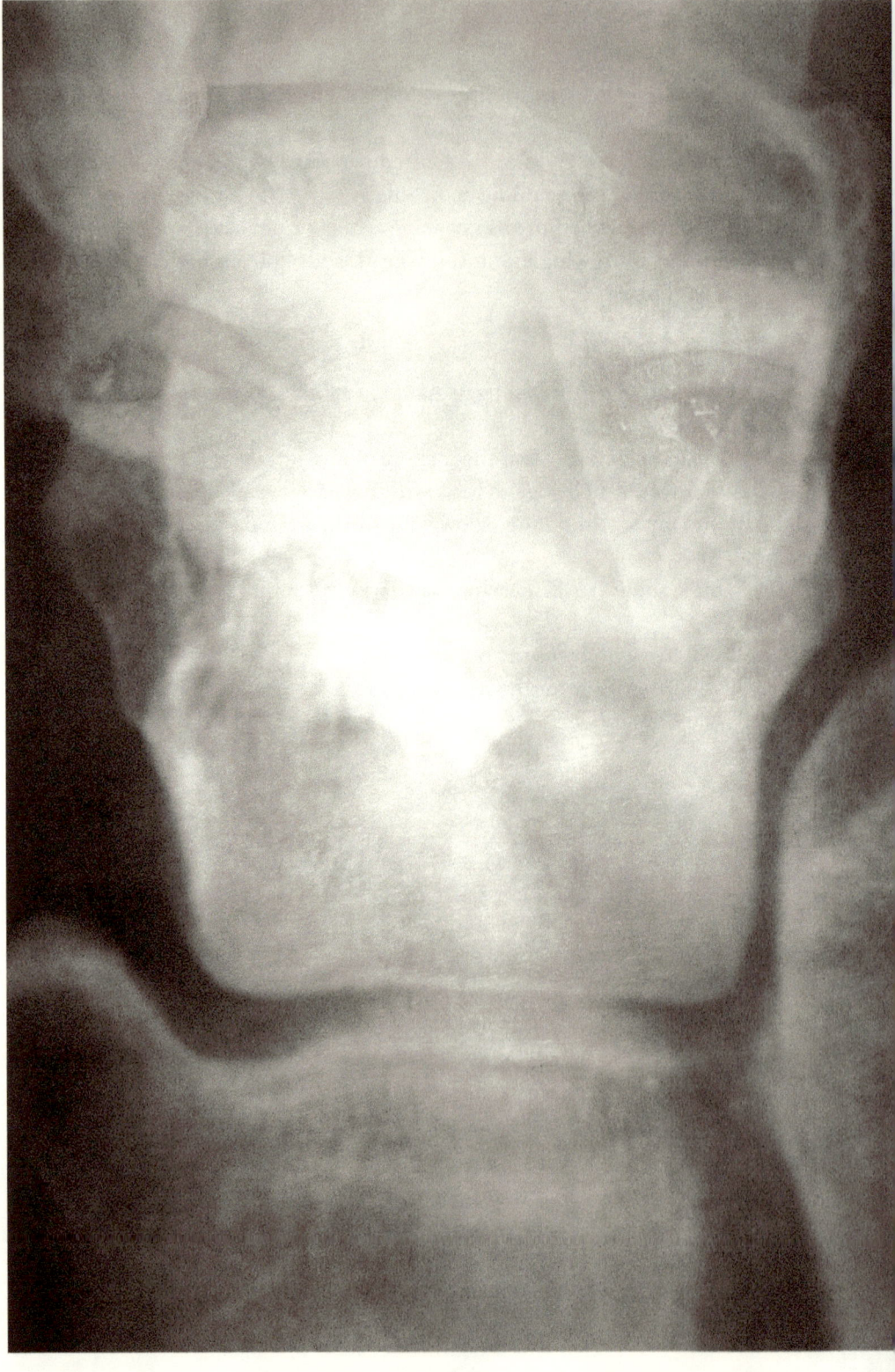

VII
CHANGING PLACES

EVELYN SHARENOV

COLLATERAL DAMAGE

The cool quiet of my car was blessed solitude before my workday. The drive to Portland began in darkness and silence. I didn't turn on the radio—just listened to the roads and freeways. Although it was still warm, day and night moved toward the balance of September's equinox. By the time I walked onto the ward, bright sunlight filtered through Lexan windows onto worn hospital carpet.

Which is to say that *that* September 11th started pretty much like any other September 11th. Most of my patients were just coming to life.

By the time they ventured from their beds and were marginally awake and dressed, I knew the rudimentary facts. In a series of coordinated suicide attacks, two jets pierced the World Trade Center's twin towers in New York City, a third crashed into the Pentagon and a fourth was down in rural Pennsylvania.

I obeyed the human imperative to call family in New York, but the lines were down or busy or there was no one there to pick up. A flat electronic voice politely suggested I place my call again later. The ward manager wanted to pray with me. I'm not a believer but that morning I needed a binding ritual. I went along.

In the usual scheme of things, a disheveled shuffling line of patients stopped by the clinical desk to pick up their medications on their way to the community room; then breakfast and a morning news program, followed by the first group session of the day. There was an eerie inevitability to what happened next. It would be just a moment before someone turned on the large screen television.

In the course of eight hours, we—two nurses and three therapists—watched together as an endless loop of video crazily replayed itself and the twin towers collapsed and rose and collapsed again and again in a bizarre demonstration of death and rebirth. We were mesmerized by the spectacle,

the upturned faces of New Yorkers, mouths open to receive burnt offerings—
the ashes of family and friends.

The most delusional patients incorporated the television images into
their illness; they smelled burned flesh and heard screams that we refused to
imagine. They watched without the filters we took for granted.

A young man saw something I could not.

"There, watch, that body exploding."

He sat up close to the television, close enough to distort any coherent
image. His hair wound into a dozen or so thick blond Rasta plaits. Dark
stubble sprouted like new mown lawn on his drawn cheeks and his arms and
legs were dotted with old or healing needle marks.

He'd been studying literature and philosophy at a small private
college in Portland, the domain of the scions of educated well-to-do parents
or talent large enough to earn a free pass. His heroin use masked the terrifying
paranoia and auditory hallucinations of his psychosis. He was here in the
middle of his first relapse—after he decided to stop his medications: he'd felt
fine, he wanted to lose the weight he'd gained from his pills, he had a new
girlfriend, he wanted to fuck, fuck, fuck. All perfectly normal desires, except
the medicines interfered with all that, disrupted everything, not just his
delusions. He'd been a junior when he stopped taking them and embarked
on what would probably be a lifelong struggle with paranoid schizophrenia.

Another man, this one middle-aged, put his arm around his college-
aged peer. His face fell into friendly creases and jowls and he was protective,
coming through a vegetative depression—the kind of smothering mood
disorder that holds you to your bed. With the help of ECT—electroconvulsive
therapy—and medication, he was fully awake. His hairline retreated, the
remainder grayed, ambivalent on how to grow old, but he was clear-eyed and
animated. His relentless depression, now lifted, provided new insight. The
two men shared a room and were fast friends. They sat together at meals and
in groups. The older man attempted to impart wisdom that had eluded him
in his own life: you have to take your meds.

Both men—in fact most of the male patients—wore athletic shoes
without shoelaces, ward policy. During groups, a row of shoe tongues lolled
to the side like panting dogs. This morning no one left the community
room to wash or dress; pajamas and bad breath were the order of the day.
Schizophrenia and major depression were untidy illnesses, and more so on
September 11th.

"How do we know the attacks are over?" one woman asked. Her visit had been preceded by a suicide attempt. A double mastectomy, chemo and radiation damaged that part of her reptilian brain devoted to survival. She was in her fifties, with disheveled gray hair. A bright purple blouse fluttered to her waist like a deflated foil birthday balloon. Residual glue from the ECT electrodes stuck to her temples and tufts of hair stuck to the glue. She huddled her forlorn body into a chair. We were supposed to help her feel safe. "What if they bomb us here?"

"How do we know this is real?"

"Yeah, what if they staged it?"

They looked to us for answers and while it seemed unlikely that terrorists had much interest in Portland, Oregon, none of us felt safe. We did, however, know it was real and had nothing to offer except words—soothing but hollow, words that didn't reflect our internal landscapes, our churning dread and apprehension.

The attacks resonated with my own terror of being trapped on an airliner that was going down, and my fears went back to my childhood. In third grade we trained to 'take cover' during air raid drills. It was cold down there on the floor under our small desks, but not as cold as the Cold War. The desks were barely wide enough to contain our length, scalp to feet. We covered our heads with our arms and tucked our legs up under our bodies. I was young, but not so young as to believe that this would help if an atom bomb fell on us. Depending on what we were made of—brick, glass, flesh—and how far we were from ground zero, we would incinerate, liquefy or vaporize.

Sometime that afternoon, my father called. I kept him in a nursing home in Portland, as if I owned him and had that right. In the twilight of our relationship, he was hobbled by dementia and didn't remember how to use the remote control or how to end a phone conversation. He was a captive audience. He wept about the city we knew so well we could walk its streets in our dreams and never get lost. I called the nursing station and asked them to hang up my father's phone and turn off his television. Other than that morning he'd been doing well, the charge nurse told me.

When I left the ward that afternoon, a hunger overwhelmed me. I wanted to hold tight to something innocent, a void so young and pure it was untouched by breath or fingertip; it had no history, no double helix, no DNA. What I did was visit my father.

The next morning everyone was haggard. The emergency room had filled and emptied and filled again during the night. We had no empty beds. Disturbed sleep and dark dreams prevailed. The hospital ramped up staffing as aftershocks shifted our roots from shared foundations—the common expectation of safety on our own soil. The first group on the first morning after nine-eleven tallied nightmares—a ground-zero litany for the mentally ill:

"My house crumbled with me in it. I was buried alive."

"I was on fire."

"A baby floated through the air toward me. It had no arms or legs."

"I had to jump out of a window but I woke up before I hit the ground."

In the big picture, I was a bit player, an editor in the narrative versions of their lives. I entered in the middle of the story, did a brief cut-and-paste, and moved on. My tools were limited: medication and conversation, as much art as science. I was a conduit: the scalpel, the IV bag, the splint that held the fractured psyche together until the crisis passed and the patient could stand on his own.

And there was always this question: what separated us from them, staff from patients? Any answer anchored in hard science was a long way off. Other than that, there were different answers on different days. On some days what separated us was a matter of degree. Anyone who experienced the loss of a parent or child or job, a life-threatening illness, the turmoil of divorce, knew how fragile sanity seemed at times, and rested well when the chill of danger passed. One morning you woke up and understood you had averted disaster.

I knew I would likely not experience the horrors that brought men and women to the ward, because whatever trigger, genetic marker or errant DNA, whatever neurotransmitter in whatever area of the brain did this to them, did not do it to me. Whether by luck or design, I remained upright. My patients were not that fortunate.

The emotional and physical boundaries that were essential on September 10th meant less on September 11th. On September 10th, the physicians, nurses and therapists on the ward had the power to say who was mad. It was easy—anyone who slept on this thirty-bed ship of fools was mad. What separated us on September 11th was just this: precious little. For a brief period of time, shared disaster obliterated the biological and cultural contexts of mental illness. What we had in common was greater than what distinguished us from each other. Jets crashed into the familiar landscape of my childhood and carefully established roles changed, patients and staff coalesced, one superimposed on the other.

On September 10th sanity was a worldview, a consensus. Madness required witnesses. On September 11th we were all witnesses, sane or mad.

At this writing, six September 11ths have come and gone. Life has moved on and away for those of us who shun the political drama and morally confused pageantry of what is now a more private sorrow.

On another brilliantly clear, splendidly warm day in Portland, in another clinical setting, it was September 11th again. A young man entered my office. There were outward signs that he took antipsychotic medication: tremors, fatigue, a broad abdomen, but vestiges of the handsome boy remained. Although he was making progress toward his goals, this morning he was sweating profusely and hypervigilant. He startled when my phone rang. Then he requested a 'prn'—a medication that could be dispensed as needed to treat transient symptoms of anxiety or agitation.

"It's September 11th," he said. On the television in the day room, another group of patients watched the towers fall.

MAXINE SUSMAN

BEFORE DINNER DRINKS

They'd sit in the gold living room chairs,
lamp between, sipping Canadian Club,
talking in low voices a mumbo-jumbo
of hemoglobin, blood count, EKG,
a code more secret than Yiddish
as if they went on private rounds
each evening without us,

confiding the day's revelations
of other men's and women's bodies
examined behind separate doors
in the office beneath their bedroom.

Years later he leaves Montefiore
after weeks of increasingly useless chemo.
She's been diagnosed with tumors
in both breasts. She asks, pleads,

Ben, what should I do? What should I do?
He can't rouse from the stupor
of lymphoma to answer.

A day post-op she waits in Beth Israel
for his brief visit. He endures our help
with clothes, stairs, the journey to the car,
the drive to the City, we wheel him down
an endless corridor to her room.
She hears him cry *Carol!* before he sees her—

they'll have one more night together
in their bed at home.

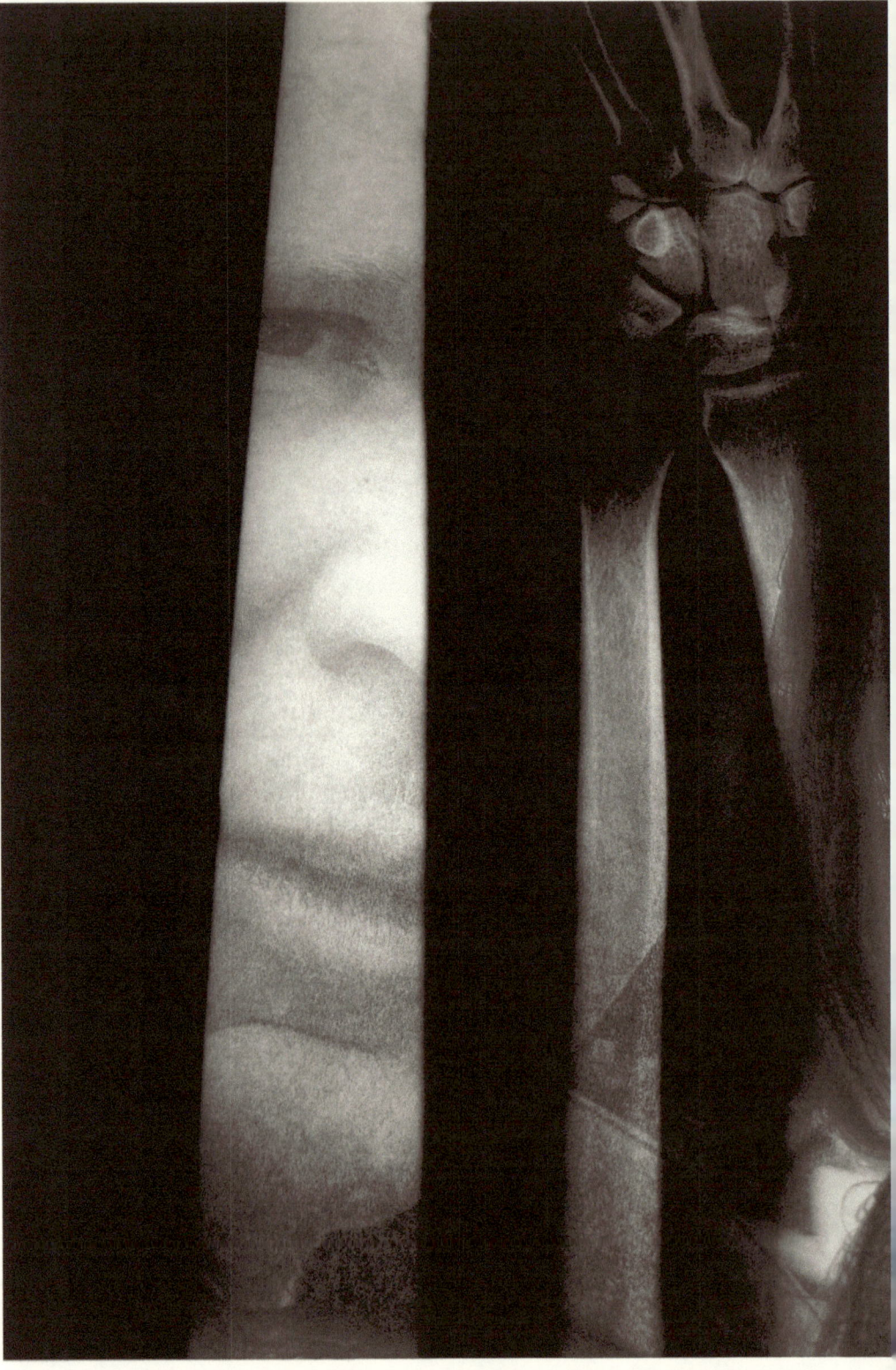

TERRY SANVILLE

IN THE WAITING ROOM

When I entered the urology clinic, the big guy was slumped in the corner chair, snores fluttering his white walrus mustache. In the full room, men stared into space while their wives paged through dog-eared editions of *Time* or *Futures Magazine*. After signing in, I took the last empty seat next to the walrus. Burbling sounds rumbled inside him and he stopped breathing. I watched his chest. It didn't move. In a panic, I reached over to nudge him. But he let out a gasp and shook himself awake.

"You okay?" I asked.

"What did you say?" He struggled to sit up. Pain creased his face.

"You weren't breathing. For a moment I was worried."

"Oh, yeah. It used to scare the dickens out of my wife when that happened. Don't worry, son, it's nothing serious." He patted my arm with a liver-spotted hand, then settled back. "You here to see Dr. Asari?"

"Ah, yes. Are you a patient of his?"

"For ten years." His grin exposed gold-capped teeth. "Has he told you yet?"

"Told me?"

"Yes, told you. You can tell by watching the guys coming out. Here comes one now."

A door leading to the examination rooms opened and a middle-aged man appeared, followed by a woman with tear-streaked cheeks. The guy looked at us with glassy eyes.

The walrus whispered, "See, he was just told."

"Christ, it doesn't look good."

"No, it doesn't. I've been watching that door for years, ever since my surgery."

I nodded and studied my hands. The waiting room gurgled with the sound of cascading water from a fountain that looked like black rain running down wrinkled glass. A nurse called a name, her voice like a songbird, rising and falling, out of place in that closed room.

"That's Kayla," the walrus said. "She was here when they told me, a good kid."

"So . . . so how long have you had cancer?"

"Ah, there's the word nobody wants to say aloud."

"Yes, the Big C."

"Good for you to get it out there. My wife and I used to dilly-dally around, as if saying it would make it worse. What about you? You have a wife?"

I shook my head. "Only an ex . . . not somebody I'd bring to this place."

"So you've had the biopsy?"

"Yes, last week. Hurt like a son-of-a-bitch."

"That's funny, I hardly felt anything. Maybe being an old fart helped."

He chuckled and nudged my arm. I tried to smile but my face felt stiff as leather. The door opened again and a man in a velour running suit came out, smiling broadly. He stopped at the counter to talk with Kayla. His voice cracked with excitement.

"This place is like Greek theater," the walrus said. "You know, the smiling and frowning masks. Nothing much in between."

"No, I suppose not."

Mr. Velour collected his paperwork and grinned. "Thanks, and I hope ta never to see y'all again."

The nurses behind the counter laughed. Some of the wives looked up from their reading, their faces frozen in what looked like hope or envy.

"That's the smiling mask we all want to wear," the walrus murmured. "But it doesn't matter."

"What the hell do you mean, it doesn't matter?" My voice came out too loud and I drew stares from other patients. I would soon learn if I had a disease that could shorten or end my life and that geezer was saying it didn't matter? He must have noticed my annoyance.

"Look, I've had surgery, then radiation. Neither of them worked and I'm headed for high-dose chemotherapy. Sure, I would have liked more time. But the amount I have left is less important than how well I spend it."

"So you hang around waiting rooms and dispense folksy advice?" I shot back, mad at his simplistic answer.

"Something like that," he said. "I didn't mean to upset you. But even if you're handed the frowning mask, you can still savor the time you have—'live life to the lees' as the poets say."

"Yes, I suppose you're right. But I was going for quality *and* quantity."

"I hope you get both. The survival rate is high if they catch it early." The walrus leaned back in his chair and closed his dark eyes. In a moment his fluttering snores returned.

The minutes passed slowly and I tried not to watch the door and the men's faces as they came out. I thought about what I would do if I got bad news. How I could squeeze the last bit of joy out of whatever time I had left. How well I would wear whatever mask I was given.

The waiting room emptied. Finally, Kayla approached and stood in front of the walrus. She leaned forward and shook him gently.

"Doctor Abrams, we're ready for you."

He groaned and pushed himself up, brushing aside her attempts to help him. Rubbing his eyes, he glanced at all the empty chairs, then at me. His grin returned.

"Live long and prosper," he said and flashed me the Vulcan salute from *Star Trek*. "My grandkids *really* like that one."

I listened to his laughter and Kayla's songbird voice as the door closed behind them.

PAULA SERGI

SURVEY

Thank you for taking the time to enter your feedback about your experience with our clinic. Your participation will help us better serve our patients.

When the doctor finally came in, he was wearing a houndstooth suit; not the traditional black and grey pattern, like in the photo of my father as a young man, but in browns and tans. I'd never seen anything quite like it. Perfectly pressed. How much would a suit like that cost? And he wore it well, a tall man, olive complexion.

James knew the way to the clinic. That's one of the things I admire about him. He can drive through traffic in LA and Chicago. Plus he speaks Italian, beautifully, even after all these years. To Italians he sounds like an American. To me, he sounds beautifully fluent. Driving in Milwaukee was a piece of cake for James. And the parking was easy—just circling and circling up until we were exposed to whatever snow might fall that day.

But the waiting room was crowded, and there was a man in a wheelchair. I'd keep those patients in another waiting area. I wondered if we were in the right place. Because there were posters about a meeting for people with MS: how to deal with the cognitive disability, the memory loss. And an announcement about being in a trial study. If I ever had a disease like that I'd want to be in a trial; not for the free meds, not for the side effects, just for the excitement of it, the eventual results, the pure science of things. Proving something beyond doubt. Even if it does take years.

The physician's assistant (who comes in to do all the work a doctor will later repeat) wore a lab coat over black slacks. The slacks fit well but were not wool; I think some kind of blend. But a tie, which is a nice touch when you're feeling apprehensive, which I will admit I was. First the right side of my body had gone numb, and now my left foot. I was tingling. And the metaphor that came to mind was that I was disappearing from the toes up. Like special effects, where you can still hear the person talking but the body isn't there. Kevin Bacon did that once.

The physician's assistant spoke like he was raised in the Midwest. But it was shocking, humiliating, really and maybe this part of the exam should be dropped. Try as I did, I could not close my eyes and touch my nose with my right hand. I hit my cheekbone once, then the other side of my face. When the doctor finally came in, he repeated this test. Again I made an ass of myself. My face, somewhere, lips once, but no nose. Did they think I was faking the first two times?

"We brought our own films," James said, as if this was a film festival. We all understood it was an MRI. But only the radiologists and the man in the houndstooth suit and his sidekick in a white lab coat could go and look at them while James and I waited in the exam room where my socks were off for a neuro check and my feet were cold. Let the patients keep their socks on.

Finally the houndstooth man came back, confident. "Let's look at your films," he said, jauntily. He spoke with an accent, like the support people you get when you call for technical support. India?

"Here we see your brain. Nothing there." But I knew what he meant. I've always been the smart one. My older sister the pretty one, my younger sister the baby, petite and lovely but naive. I'm the intelligent one, a master's degree and love reading, writing thesis papers, developing a thesis. So I know he didn't mean 'nothing' there. I know he meant no lesions.

"See these two small areas in the spinal chord?" He pointed with his pen. "Well the quality of this film isn't the best. They're gray, little cloud tufts. Here we have it. Here we have the reason for the numbness on your right side . . ."

Houndstooth in winter. Perfectly pressed. Fits him to a tee. The length of the pants just right. James's father was a tailor; James knows suits. It kills him to see the wrong length of pant, cheap material. When I went back to the west coast for a conference, I met with my former boyfriend. He was still so nice, so witty and funny. Still called me by my pet name. Thinks I talk like the people in Fargo. But his pants—all wrong. That's the first time I realized how much of James had gotten into me—the pants were corduroy, for Christ sake, and there was a matching jacket—such a bad idea. Not since the leisure suit had a look been so wrong. I was impressed with his effort; it was sort of a suit but casual enough to wear in a city where everyone hikes. Probably the best sales in any REI anywhere. Just not a look he, or anyone, could pull off.

But this man in the houndstooth, he could look into my brain and come up with a diagnosis in a minute. Actually, less.

And then there was a lot of talk about the drugs that could be used, and I nodded a lot. I mean, all the signs were there, but absent a good film, I was still enchanted by door number one: the viral theory. My best friend liked door number one, too, and she is a nurse and very smart.

They gave me a choice: a spinal tap or another MRI. Hmm, let me think about it a minute: spinal taps are said to be very painful. Everyone says that except the neurologist. The worst part is staying still while the needle is inserted into the spinal cord and the potential for a bad, bad, headache after. I call it invasive. The needle. The headache.

Or, my second option, another MRI, where you lie perfectly still while they slide you into a tube and send rattling noises into your brain. I've always been very smart, even in grade school. The teachers liked me, used my homework as an example. Only Mary Lou was smarter and a boy named Thomas but I'm talking about the girls now and some years Mary Lou was in another class so she didn't matter. I chose the tube and the bullet sounds toward the brain because I'd just had four of those and now felt like a pro. I can lie very still for those and if my feet are warm, I do quite well. The X-ray techs have praised me. How do I do it? Imagery, of course. You think those years of yoga didn't count towards anything? I can imagine myself lying on a warm beach, the waves crashing upon the shore, though it's been years since I actually did lie on a warm beach with waves crashing.

My attorney boyfriend, who did not do a lot of hiking, had a deal on a timeshare and invited me along. I shouldn't say boyfriend, because, after six months of dating, I discovered that he never had the *mens rea* for monogamy. He didn't like me that way. We could spend every night of the week together, but it did not imply any kind of reciprocal commitment. But that trip to Molokai, the waves, the warm sand. He was tall, probably six-foot three, and could wear a suit well. But I only saw him in a suit once, and I think it was gray. Gray means never having to make a decision.

And a couple of years later James and I had a belated honeymoon on the Big Island. I dug a little hole on the beach and let my five-month pregnant belly rest in the sand. That's why our son has such wanderlust, the sound of the waves. Almost twenty-five years ago.

But the beach is not the image I go for when I'm in the tube. My secret is this: a poem by Sharon Olds about how she wrapped her daughter in a blanket. A cocoon. All mothers wrap their babies in a blanket; that's how they feel secure. But Sharon Olds did it for her daughter when she was older, maybe ten. And the daughter took delight in it. I have done the very same thing for my boys, and they laughed and laughed. Something about pretending to be all caught up, like in a spider's web, but knowing all along your mother will free you when you've had enough. I wrapped my little sister like that when I was taking care of her. She laughed and laughed.

Of course I opted for the MRI. I was feeling disoriented; where is the lab in this huge building? Why are they handing me a key to a locker when my hand does not work, will not obey, will not open a locker or the buttons on my blouse?

The X-ray tech, who was wearing blue scrubs, asked if I could hold still, if I was claustrophobic. I told him I'd be his best patient ever, he'll see. "All I need is my feet covered with a blanket, and a folded wash cloth over my eyes." He started an IV in my right hand, at my suggestion because I can't feel it anyway. His nametag said Jamal. His hands were dark, shiny almost, and the contrast with the blue scrubs was nice. All I needed, I reminded the tech, as he began to walk away into his own room where a tinny voice announces every so often you're doing fine, just seven more minutes . . . the next scan will last eleven . . . was the call button.

Jamal got me the call button and apologized for forgetting it. "And you'd be like 'Yeah I needed you but you didn't leave me the call button and now I hate you.'" It was funny. He was the funniest tech I've had so far. He made me smile through the bullet sounds to the head, and in my new cocoon the minutes passed. I tried to sleep, but that didn't happen. Instead, the images that came to me were brown and blue, tree branches and sky. How corny was it that his name was so common, for a black man, I mean? How funny that the first three letters were the same as my husband's name?

After the procedure, where I hardly moved at all, if at all, I told him my secret: about the cocoon and the poem and my imagery. He thought that was pretty good. He wished all his patients could lie that still. "I finally found something I'm good at," I joked with Jamal, because he had made me laugh so I wanted to make him laugh. And he did. A real belly laugh.

"I'm sure you're good at other things, too," he said. I told him it also helped to have a good tech, one who you know is watching from the far away room. One who can share a joke.

"That's interesting," he said. "Yesterday I was told I was a lousy X-ray tech. Some guy really chewed my ass." Now don't record that Jamal said the word "ass" with a patient. I had opened the door to colloquial talk with my own casual use of language.

"People are just scared when they're here," I said. "That's why they say things like that and blame you. They're scared and freaking out."

"But there's no reason to be rude." I agreed with him.

"It bothered me all night," he said. "After I went home, I still felt bad, all night." I wondered if the doctor or even the physician's assistant would think about me after they got home. I wondered if Jamal would think of me tonight.

Jamal said, "You just made my day. So why you here?"

"I have MS," I said. The words sounded wrong, like they came from the far away tech's room, all wrong like my wooden hand trying to tie my shoes, but it was good practice. "Just found out about an hour ago."

"Ah, well, you know what? They have so many new treatments and meds out for that now, you gonna be all right." And he touched my shoulder. I suppose a X-ray tech shouldn't do that. I hope you don't mention anything about this on his evaluation.

And though James was waiting for me upstairs, and he knew the way home, and he has always been a wonderful husband, I wanted to go home with Jamal that night. Because he speaks my language. We'd talk about his day at work, and we'd laugh.

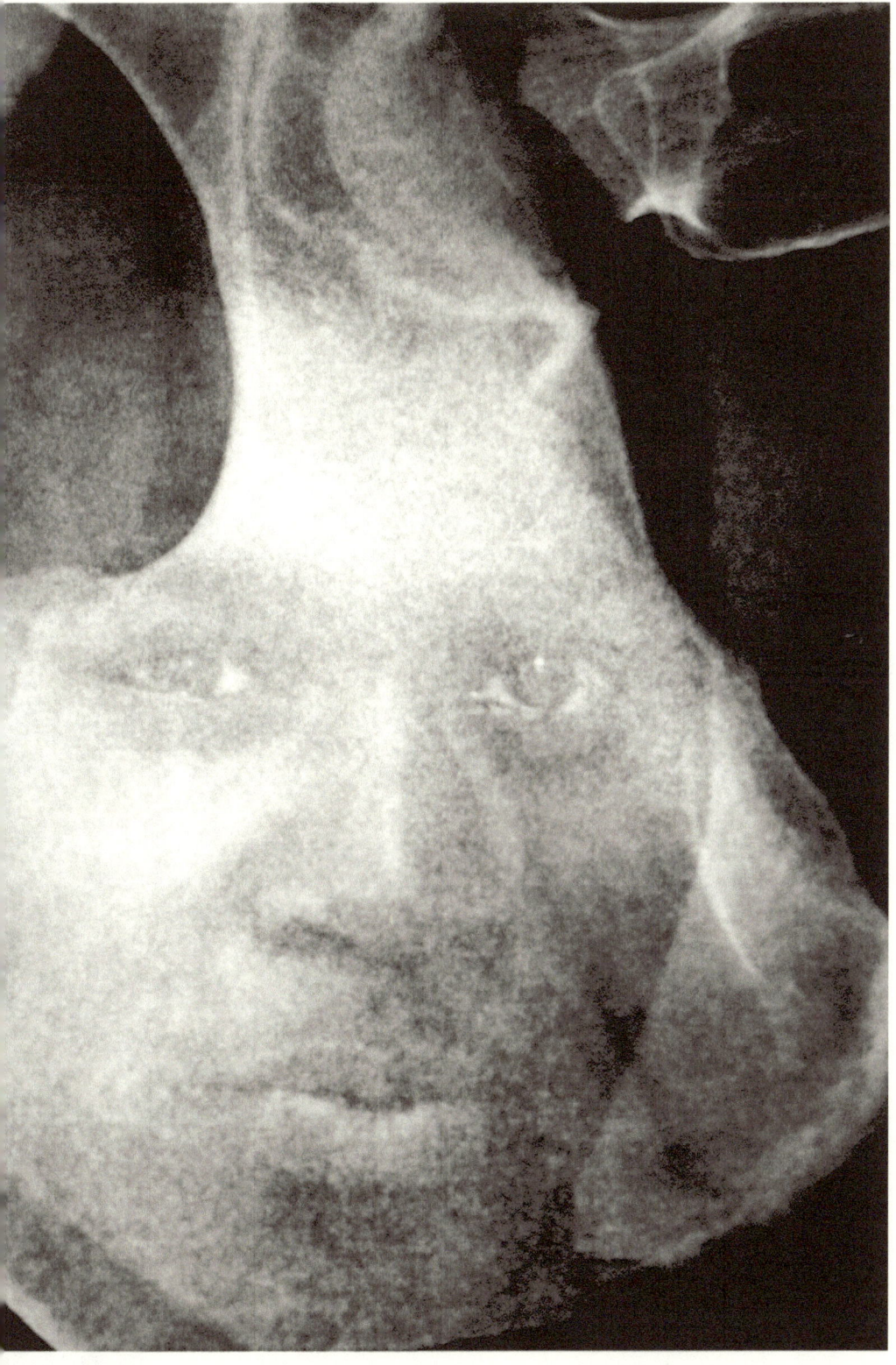

NINA GABY
(*Scribe*)

WHAT MATTERS AND WHAT WE MIGHT WANT TO FORGET

We live in a world filled with language. Language imparts identity, meaning, and perspective to our human community. Just as the language of power and greed has the potential to destroy us, the language of reason and empathy has the power to save us. Writers can inspire a kinder, fairer, more beautiful world, or incite selfishness, stereotyping, and violence. Writers can unite people or divide them.
Mary Pipher, *Writing to Change the World.*

Introduction:

The "Situation and the Story" is what we call our therapy group at Second Spring, a rural, recovery-based facility in central Vermont where fourteen residents live while transitioning from the state psychiatric hospital to the community. Second Spring is alternatingly described as "bucolic and relaxed with a home-like atmosphere" to "boring as hell."

Our program blends the Medical Model of psychiatric care with Recovery Principles of peer support, self-determination and individuality. The "Situation and the Story" (the title is borrowed from a book by Vivian Gornick that our facilitator has used in group) is the second step of our Cognitive-Behavioral Therapy, where we as a group take our situations and see if by rewriting them, if by changing the language, we can modify our emotions and consequently influence our behavior and choices in the future. We also hope, as writers, to inspire.

Our group describes itself:

Anonymous contributors: two females, four males
Mark: currently sober forty-seven-year-old white male with PTSD and
        Major Depressive Disorder
Charles: forty-six-year-old Caucasian male with Schizoaffective Disorder
        and a few challenging behavioral issues
Wilhelm: thirty-five-year-old human being
Adelit: forty-one-year-old Recovery Worker
Dr. R: resident in Psychiatry
Nina: sixty-year-old Advanced Practice Registered Nurse and Clinical
        Director
Gabrielle: female Recovery Worker
Female Case Manager

The idea for this essay came from visiting the UniversalTable.org website while reading a piece that our Clinical Director, the group facilitator, had published. Both the clinicians and the residents of the facility could relate to the essay she wrote about a patient she would never forget. We talked about the emergence of 'medical narrative' and how the act of writing not only educates others but helps us to change how we feel by the act of expression. Individually we did not feel as if we were professional enough as writers but felt that as a group, with well over three hundred years between us either as clinicians or consumers, we have the expertise to address the question: "For Better or For Worse, the Doctor or Nurse We Will Never Forget."

Our process first took us to groups focused on brainstorming. The brainstorming process led us to explore a number of avenues, some painful, but all leading to the conclusion that none of us had one single person we would never forget, but a collective. We looked at the systems that have influenced our recovery, systems created by individuals and their unique interweaving into our lives. At the table in our conference room sat the residents of the facility, carrying a variety of diagnoses of major mental illness. Also present were Recovery staff with an assortment of backgrounds. One staff in particular had escaped great violence in his homeland and provides quiet proof of hope every day for those around him. Another, a case manager who began as a peer support staff bravely talked of her own experiences "on both sides of the coin." The

Clinical Director, an Advanced Practice Registered Nurse, facilitated the group and wrote the final draft of this essay. A young psychiatrist in training joined us every Thursday to further his understanding of treatment and recovery.

We met twice a week. Our dialogue followed emotionally descriptive and thought-provoking paths. Despite the symptoms that periodically interfered, or maybe in great part because of them, we worked hard. We brainstormed themes. We thought about whom we might never forget. What have we learned—what can we teach? These are the themes and the stories we came up with:

Who is the expert?

> *"I am the expert on myself, but I know I am not the only expert."*
> —Anonymous

If we look at those we can't forget in terms of those who provide care, we might be tempted to view them as the experts. From our discussions we realized that while there were many with expertise, those we remember are those who either were most caring or those who were not.

We also concluded that 'expertise' is a collaborative process. The Mental Health Recovery Model is different than the traditional Medical Model in that in Recovery we conceptualize this collaboration as acknowledging that the patient is the expert on her or himself.

> *"I know what's wrong, I go for help in how to fix it."* —Anonymous

> *"You know the most about yourself. I am the expert on myself. Nobody did it for me. It came from my desire to get better."* —Charles

That being said, most of the group acknowledged that being heard and being cared for were important, especially when someone is their most vulnerable. Psychiatric decompensation is such a time, and this is also a time when the power differential can be very frightening.

"Sometimes doctors have a god complex." —Anonymous

"Sometimes they are overly aggressive (doctors). Verbally and physically. But sometimes they come around." —Anonymous

"Sometimes the social worker stands between me and the doctor." —Anonymous

"Are you kidding? I was glad the social workers were between me and the doctors." —Anonymous

The mental health system is made up of many disciplines, and despite the often minimal contact people have with an actual MD, it is the doctor that often gets the most blame or the most credit. In an early group, participants spoke of the times they have been under-treated or poorly treated in emergency rooms or at community mental health centers when they have recognized that they were in need of help. We utilized the group to role-play how a good visit should go and to explore when a visit went bad. One participant talked openly of his decompensation and the perceived lack of attention he received from his team, resulting in threats of violence towards his doctor and eventual hospitalization. This is a young man who states with angry sarcasm that this is certainly someone he will never forget.

On the other hand, another participant, Mark, credits both doctors and a social worker with saving his life. His primary care physician responded on a Sunday to abnormal lab work, a dangerously high potassium level that could have resulted in death. The physician contacted us and we worked together to get the resident into the Emergency Room and the ICU in near record time. The social worker that he will never forget taught him an invaluable method of relaxation, an intervention that he uses to this day. Our Medical Director at Second Spring, along with our past Program Director, believed in him enough to change our admission criteria so he could begin again here in this environment. It is profound for him the realization that if he were still in jail or even in the state hospital, all these life-saving measures may not have been possible.

So we looked next at the process of 'life-saving measures' and how they sometimes happen.

Involuntary holds

> *"What does it matter to society if someone kills themselves?"*
> —Charles
> *"Why can't people have the choice to neglect themselves?"*
> —Anonymous
> *"Whether it's voluntary or involuntary, what is the overall benefit?"*
> —Adelit
> *"What benefits the community?"*
> —Case manager

Mental Health Law in Vermont allows licensed psychiatrists and other physicians working in concert with qualified mental health professionals to hold a person with dangerous psychiatric symptoms for a period of evaluation. Depending on further determination by the psychiatric team, a person may be confined to the hospital and possibly be placed on court ordered medications against their will. The Clinical Director who has worked in emergency departments and on crisis teams feels she has saved lives by having patients held in the safety of a hospital until the crisis has passed.

> *"People have come to me later, sometimes years later, to thank me for making a decision when they were not capable themselves."* —Nina, Clinical Director

Being in a position of power as one is when making decisions to hold one against their will is a profound responsibility, one that the person being held does not forget.

> *"I was a blank canvas with colors pouring out of me like a sieve. I think they wanted to save me and I had to depend on them for every element . . . they saw how vulnerable a person could be."* —Mark

Nor does the person making the decision.

> *"The least favorite part of my job, which sometimes affects my sleep, is when I have to decide whether to lock someone up versus letting them*

go. I have to be prepared to go to court to defend either decision."
—Dr. R.

Fear exploits, the group concurs. Being involuntarily held is detrimental to one's fiber, one's dignity.

"The trauma . . . even today it carries into my life." —Anonymous

Ah, but is always "for worse"?

"It was a decision made by the 'experts'. I didn't like it but they had to. I was threatening to the public." —Charles

"At the time I was upset that I was committed, but it was good to have the medical attention, get my diabetes figured out. I didn't have anyplace to go. The hospital was a place to go." —Anonymous

"Usually people don't just go from zero to ten. Instead of involuntary status I should have gotten more support out in the community from professionals. It could have been handled differently." —Wilhelm

And how do people view those who have gone through this? "On-lookers, they are like paparazzi, pests," one participant quipped. We wonder, what do people think when they see someone become mentally ill? Science views mental illness as a function of brain dysregulation, an organic lack of balance, much like diabetes.

But how do people view themselves?

Research bears out that those with a mental illness are no more violent than those presumably sane. However, the road back to self-acceptance takes time after an exacerbation. With time people can view their helpers with better equanimity.

"I was in the criminal justice system because of what happened when I went off my meds. If it weren't for my lawyer, she got the judge to review the findings of the doctor who interviewed me before the trial. The judge

was just ready to try me. But she got him to wait for the results of the forensic psychiatrist and he finally agreed I was insane during the event. So I was treated for a disorder instead of being put on trial for my crimes. It's like finding that fine line between the two . . . being called 'insane' or being labeled a 'criminal.' It's a paradox and either way you feel sick. If you are a criminal it's not good in society. On the other hand, oh my god, 'I'm insane' and how do I ever go about making decisions for myself? Today I am lucid, clear thinking, and three-quarters on my way to being autonomous. I still don't have total freedom but I am receiving treatment and taking advantage of the opportunities. And you know what? The labels don't have the power they used to have." —Charles

We can add lawyers to the list of those who may never be forgotten.

Summary:

"It's not a storybook ending." —Anonymous

"We made it through the process. Whether you admire us or look down on us, we are better people for what we have been through."
—The Group

Group work is about process. The renowned writer, analyst and researcher, Irvin Yalom, MD, identifies eleven factors as the basis for why we even have group psychotherapy at all. The complex process of change is achieved through what Yalom identifies as the "intricate interplay of human experiences," which he calls the Therapeutic Factors. Among them:

• Instillation of hope
• Universality
• Altruism
• Imparting information
• Development of socialization skills
• Interpersonal learning
• Group cohesiveness
• Existential Factors

Our group affiliation allows us to achieve these for ourselves. In the act of writing, we impart this information to others. No, certainly there is no storybook ending that has been made possible by a doctor, a nurse, a lawyer, a therapist. No magical single pill.

But have we been successful? During our planning we became cohesive in our intent, during our brainstorming we realized we were not alone. During our writing we became bored with the editing and re-editing process but learned that we can tolerate boredom and we learned about the interpersonal learning and socialization that takes place as we plod on. The very act of submitting this essay for consideration of publication connects us with the larger world . . . will we be acceptable? And altruism hopefully weaves in and out as we provide each other with support and explore how to better understand our actions and the actions of those around us.

There are many we will never forget, among them, each other. Today we become writers. Today we are not mental patients or clinicians. This is our situation and this is what we make of our stories.

Resources:

Gaby, Nina. "The Inventories We Keep." *The Patient Who Changed My Life.*
    www.universaltable.org, 2009.
Gornick, Vivian. *The Situation and the Story: the art of personal narrative.*
    New York: Farrar, Strauss, Giroux, 2001.
Pipher, Mary. *Writing to Change the World.* New York: Riverhead
    Books, 2006.
Yalom, Irvin D. *Theory and Practice of Group Psychotherapy.* New York:
    Basic Books, 1970.

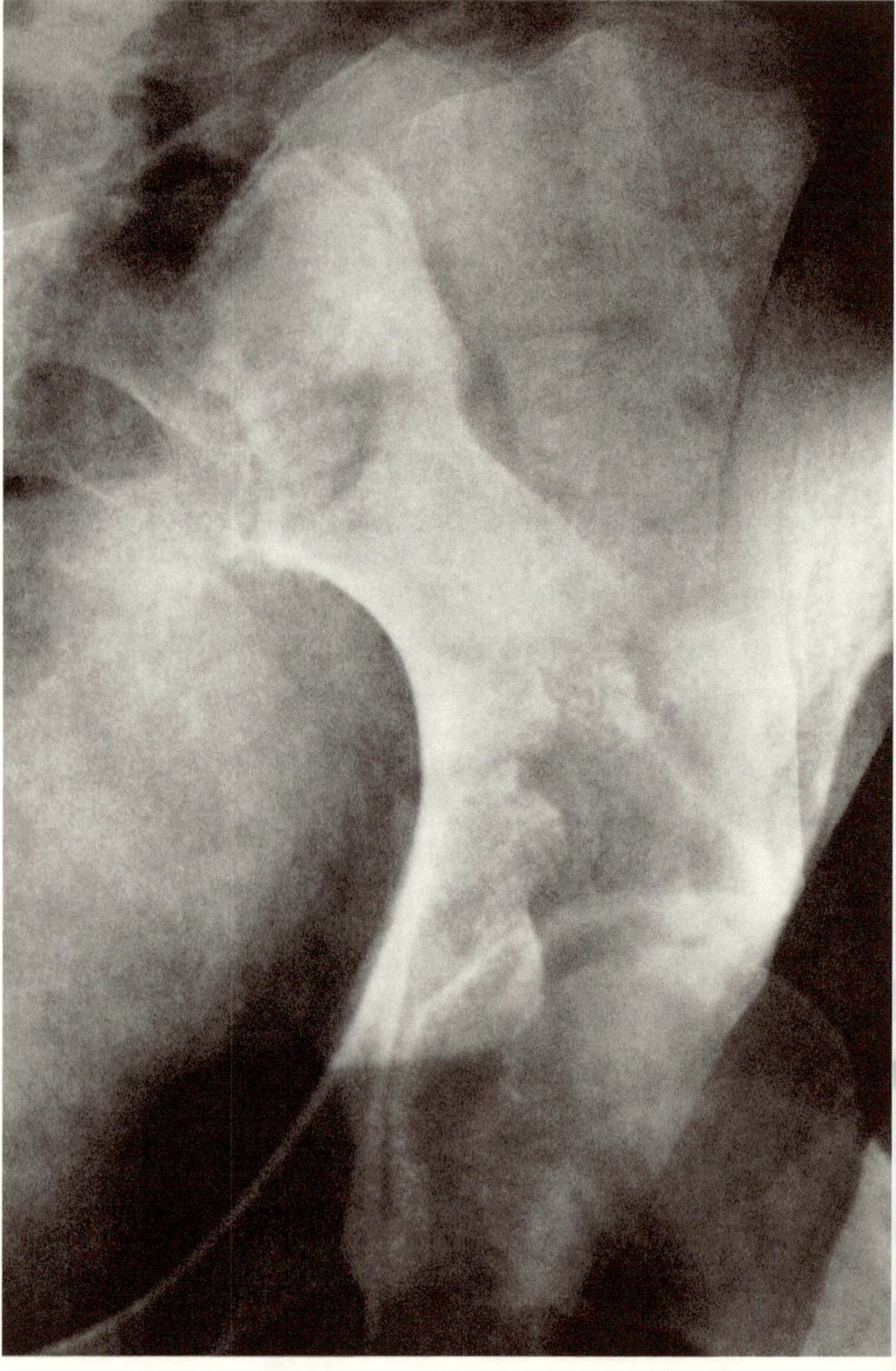

GERRI LUCE

THE FINE LINE BETWEEN LOVE AND INSANITY

I am in love with my therapist Dr. Adena. I don't only love her for all the on-target interpretations she has made or, as she would gently remind me, the work that we have accomplished together. There is, in the therapeutic community, a difference between loving one's therapist in appreciation for all she has done for you and being in love with her the way in which you would be with an intimate partner. I am a heterosexual female and so is Dr. Adena. In the analytic world, it is possible for a female analysand to fall in love with her female analyst and not be considered homosexual.

When I first started working with her more that four years ago in October of 2005, I had quit treatment with a therapist I had been seeing for thirteen years, I had stopped taking all my psychiatric medications (which for me are as critical as water). I was barely functioning at work (ironically, I am a therapist). The only treatment I was receiving was from a long-time therapy group. I was breaking down, much like the transmission on an old car that keeps stalling as its owner attempts to inch it forward.

My group therapist saw the negative spiral that had caught me in its grip and referred me to Dr. Adena for a medication consultation.

"Gerri," she said to me, "you're going to end up in the (psychiatric) hospital. Is that what you want?"

At that point I had been out of the hospital for four years—my longest stretch since my first hospitalization for anorexia in 1988. I didn't want to go back and I trusted Robin whose group I had been in for several years. Reluctantly, I made an appointment with Dr. Adena.

I don't remember most of what transpired during the ensuing months; what I do know is that I began seeing Dr. Adena, who is a psychiatrist and an analyst not only for medication but for psychotherapy. Apparently, the re-starting of treatment came too late for soon after I started seeing her I became actively suicidal and she hospitalized me. I was so severely depressed and self-destructive that I received several courses of electro-convulsive therapy (ECT) treatment, one of the most feared side effects of which is memory loss. The first six months of treatment with Dr. Adena have been erased.

What ensued was a major breakdown: six inpatient hospitalizations over a period of eighteen months, from October of 2005 to February of 2007. I lost my job and I became addicted to Klonopin (a powerful anti-anxiety medication). I snuck razor blades into the hospital during one stay and cut myself on various parts of my body.

I was a mess, a total fucked-up skeleton of a human being for the first year and a half that Dr. Adena saw me, going in and out of the hospital using it like a carousel going in endless circles. I picture the carousel as one of the ones with painted grimacing horses on it, one of the ones that scare little children and make them scream to get off. There was no possible way she could have gotten to know me with all those interruptions in the treatment, yet she stuck with me. We have a contract that she put in writing for me since she knew I wouldn't remember it because of the ECT:

1) If I cut myself, even the slightest scratch, I have to have it checked out by a (medical) physician, before I can see her again.

2) If I drop below 110 lbs. (I am 5'6" tall), I have to be admitted to the eating disorder unit of the hospital.

3) If I attempt suicide, Dr. Adena will do everything she can to save me, then she will end our treatment.

The stipulations in this contract are critical in keeping my self-destructive urges at bay, and number three, crucial in keeping my suicidal fantasies from becoming reality.

In January of 2007, Dr. Adena and a nutritionist whom I had seen only twice decided together that I needed to be admitted to an inpatient eating disorder unit. I did not weigh 110 lbs. as our contract had stipulated; I weighed 118 lbs., however I had lost twenty-four pounds in several months and was consuming a mere 250 calories per day. I was abusing laxatives and had made several trips to the emergency room for chest pains where the doctors had discovered my potassium was low. When Dr. Adena delivered the news of the impending hospitalization I was furious with her. I felt she had reneged on her part of the contract by throwing me in the hospital when my weight was clearly above our agreed upon amount. I was so ill and so into my disease that I was incapable of seeing what I was doing to myself.

When I was discharged from that inpatient unit I was sent to an outpatient eating disorder day program as subsequent follow-up treatment. As I was meeting with their psychiatrist he got off the phone after consulting with Dr. Adena, and he turned and said to me, "She really cares about you. She is committed to you." My anger at her for hospitalizing me melted. I saw it pooling on a white tile floor just like my blood did when I cut myself and it fell from my body. I wiped it up with a towel, threw it in the trash and it was gone. And I never cut myself again, though I can't say I haven't had strong urges. And I can't say I haven't bought razor blades, taken them home with me from the store and caressed the steel, feather-light blades.

In addition to my diagnoses of anorexia and depression, I was also diagnosed with borderline personality disorder (BPD), which is one of the illnesses that Dr. Adena specializes in treating. BPD is known for several distinct characteristics:

- Intense relationships with a great deal of conflict, also a strong sensitivity to a fear of abandonment.
- Difficulties related to the stability of sense of self.
- Emotional instability; feeling like we are on an emotional roller coaster with very quick shifts in mood.
- Associated with a tendency to engage in risky and impulsive behaviors; prone to engage in self-harming behaviors like cutting and suicide attempts.

In an article "Is Transference Focused Therapy for BPD (Borderline Personality Disorder) Right for You," by Kristalyn Salters-Pedneault, PhD, transference is described as

> the theoretical process by which emotions are transferred from one person to another . . . it is presumed that the patient's feelings about important people in her life (such as parents or caregivers) are transferred onto the therapist, so that she comes to feel about and reacts to the therapist as she would to these important figures in their lives. It is believed that through the transference, the therapist can see how the individual interacts with people, and the therapist uses this information to help the individual build healthier relationships.

It was incredibly difficult for me to admit my love for Dr. Adena aloud to her in the course of a forty-five minute session. I remember feeling it, viscerally, almost in a preverbal sense, before I could put it into words, not knowing, not realizing what I was experiencing because I had never felt this type of love for another person before in my lifetime. This feeling in my gut, most likely lasted for a good two years before I was able, with her encouragement, to speak the words out loud. And I could not (and cannot to this day) even say, "I love you." These words come out more as, "My love for you is . . ." or "My feelings of love for you cause me to . . . ."

These feelings are a specialized form of transference known as erotic transference. A general understanding of erotic transference is defined as a positive transference that is accompanied by sexual fantasies that the patient understands to be unrealistic.

When Dr. Adena first informed me that what I was experiencing was this 'erotic transference,' I felt intensely ashamed and humiliated, but confused. I wasn't gay and I didn't want to have sex with her. I did what I always do when a concept makes me acutely uncomfortable—I went searching for answers—this time on the internet and I googled "erotic transference female therapists and female patients."

Up came a book by Florence W. Rosiello, PhD, *Deepening Intimacy in Psychotherapy; Using the Erotic Transference and Countertransference*, with a chapter titled, "Homoerotic Transference and Countertransference between a Female Analyst and Female Patients." In it she discusses the views of a therapist, Bollas:

> [Bollas] elaborates that there is a displaced manifestation of the erotic transference in heterosexual same-sex analyses, one that could best be described as a form of 'rhapsodic identification.' In this particular relationship with the analyst, the patient falls in love with both real and imagined aspects of the analyst's character and perceived life, such as how the analyst expressed ideas, his mannerisms, or his sensitivities. 'The patient develops an intense inner relation to the object of identification that gains its rhapsodic character from the analyst's . . . presence', a type of idealized love.

When I read this, I thought I had found the answer, what I now realize was a rationalization, a postponement of the truth. I sat in Dr. Adena's office across from her and admired the way in which she wore her clothes and her subtle, but obviously expensive jewelry. I studied her long elegant fingers and carefully manicured nails. I fantasized about being a part of her life with her husband, her children and their dog, sitting in front of the fireplace in their Tudor-style home playing Scrabble.

What I didn't want was to have sex with her. I didn't have sexual fantasies that included sleeping in the same bed with her, longing for the two of us to lie together, caressing and kissing each other. The vivid picture that brought to my mind nauseated me.

Simultaneously, while this issue of erotic transference was torturing my psyche, I had begun working again as a therapist. In the midst of my multiple hospitalizations, I had received Social Security disability and was surviving on that entitlement; however, Dr. Adena's philosophy was that one should not languish on the rolls of governmental assistance indefinitely. Due to the multiple courses of ECT that I had received because of my suicidal depressions, I truly believed that my brain had been damaged at an organic level and I would never again regain the capacity to work as a therapist. In order to work effectively, I would be required to remember the patients' stories from session-to-session and I didn't believe that I would be capable of that skill.

Dr. Adena encouraged me not only with the scientific data that ECT did not cause organic brain damage, but by discussing my fantasies about what it would be like to work again, my unrealistic expectations of perfectionism and my fear of failure.

"You sit here and make these brilliant interpretations day after day," I practically accused her. "How could I ever measure up? What if I forget something important that a patient tells me between sessions? What if I have to write a session note at the end of the day and I forget what the patient said?" My fears and my lack of confidence spilled out into the air.

Dr. Adena offered some practical suggestions: "Write the note in session"—but each one was met with resistance.

"I can't do that—the patient will want to know what I'm writing." I practically hurled the words in her face. It wasn't really about the practical suggestions; she could have told me almost anything and I would have met it with an argument. I was simply terrified to return to work.

In therapy, Dr. Adena persisted, and we continued to explore the issue and the root of my fears. My mother had been a workaholic, extraordinarily successful, and I was afraid that I wouldn't measure up in her eyes even though at that point she had passed away six years before.

Toward the end of the eighteen-month span I became restless at my lack of productivity, at my boredom watching *Law and Order* reruns daily on cable television. I summoned my courage and began to search for employment. I discussed with Dr. Adena how to disguise the gap in my resume, finally settling on saying I took a break to write. At that time in my writing career, I had published several essays, so I felt justified in putting that profession on my resume.

The first several interviews were a disaster; finally in the age of online job searches, I saw a tiny ad in *The New York Times* for an outpatient mental health clinic in New York City. It would be quite a commute, parking would be a struggle but I sent my resume and was offered an interview. The director of the clinic seemed especially interested in my writing; she inquired about the subject matter and I lied (the true content of my writing consists of essays about my mental illness). I said I wrote about the course of treatment with patients; the transference, the counter-transference. I panicked when she said she would like to read them, but to-date she seems to have forgotten.

I was offered the job. It was part-time on a fee-for-service basis, which means one only gets paid for the patients actually seen. We hadn't set a start date when the director called me at home on a Wednesday afternoon and asked me if I could start the next day. Calmly I said yes, and when I got off the phone, I began to have an anxiety attack and put in an emergency call to Dr. Adena. The call was brief; she actually pointed out the benefit of not having to endure anticipatory anxiety, and when I stopped hyper-ventilating long enough to listen to what she was saying, I had to admit she was right.

One day a week turned into two days a week, which after three months turned into four days a week. At that point, the director called me into her office and informed me she would like me to start working on what is termed "Utilization Reviews." This meant that I would be reviewing the chart of every patient who had an intake interview and make the determination whether he or she is appropriate for admission. Concerns to be considered would be strong suicidal or homicidal thoughts (in which case they would be hospitalized), a history of violent acting out, and other similar issues. Dr. Adena suggested the added responsibility and trust in my judgment were like a promotion without a raise.

Over the first nine months, working four days a week, my confidence was growing slowly. I found that my memory was not as poor as I thought it was going to be and patients responded well to my therapeutic style. I was also able to discuss troubling cases with Dr. Adena and we explored how my own issues may be affecting my work with my patients.

The clinic is large and busy but they employ primarily fee-for-service clinicians like me—I think the number of full-time therapists is under ten, and the number of fee-for-service therapists (including the evening staff) is close to forty. At the nine-month point, I was in the director's office discussing another matter and I was able to choke out the words I had been silently rehearsing for the past month.

"Ellen, I just want you to know how much I like working here and if a full-time position should open up, I hope that you will consider me for it."

She looked up at me from her littered desk with her glasses down at the end of her nose and replied, "Give me a couple of weeks, I'm working on it."

I left her office not knowing what that meant. Had she already been thinking about it before I asked? Was someone leaving and was she considering me for her replacement? My anxiety and anticipation was charged when several days later she casually mentioned to me that she would like to meet with me the following week.

I talked to everyone I knew about what that meeting could possibly entail, exploring all the options, soliciting the opinions of my family and friends, and of course, Dr. Adena in the session before the weekend. The consensus was simple; either she was going to offer me a full-time position, or in the midst of the recession, she was going to say that the clinic could not currently afford to take on the salary and the benefits of another full-time staff member.

It was a Wednesday morning. I typically get into the office at 7:30 a.m., although my first patient doesn't arrive until 9 a.m. Leaving the suburb where I live so early lets me avoid the inevitable rush hour traffic. When I get to the office this early, it also gives me time to pull my charts, check my voicemail, and get things together for the day. Also if I have time, I can do paperwork like treatment plans, or the unavoidable insurance forms and get them out of the way. Ellen usually arrives around 8 a.m. She likes to empty her mailbox, have a cup of coffee and also organize herself for the day. I think I had a cancellation around ten so we arranged to meet then. She was direct:

"I'd like to offer you a full-time position here at the clinic starting the beginning of next quarter. We don't pay well but we do offer good benefits . . ." She went on to explain them and I tried hard to pay attention but I was ecstatic. Look how far I had come—and I couldn't help thinking, "I can't wait to tell Dr. Adena." My next session was Friday morning. I debated whether or not to leave a message on her voicemail. I decided I wanted to tell her in person. I wanted to see the reaction on her face, in her eyes, see what hopefully would be pleasure and pride.

I was disappointed. She is not an especially expressive person; at least not in the therapeutic session. I wonder what she is like away from the office with her family and friends. One session she came in with a cane and an air boot on her leg. She said she had broken her foot dancing at a wedding. Dr. Adena dancing! It was a picture I could not imagine. I tried to imagine what she was wearing, how high were her heels, what music was playing—was it a slow dance or rock 'n roll? But that was all she would say by way of explanation and I didn't ask any further questions.

When I told her about the full-time position, she congratulated me, then she turned it on me as she always does. How do you feel about it? What does it mean to you? I told her I couldn't have done it without her—that it had been two-and-a-half years since I had started working with her and now that I was showing signs of progress—now that I was a "well and functioning person" I was terrified she was going to declare that I didn't need to see her anymore and she would end the therapy with me. And I started to cry. And panic. And she asked me, "Can you ever imagine the day where you would feel that you wouldn't need to see me?"

And I answered with the most certainty I could muster, "No, never. I will always need you."

She reassured me. "You will be the one who will decide when you don't need to talk to me." And that made me love her even more.

The panic gradually abated. And then the session was over and it was time to leave the safety of her office, turn my world upside down and go to work where I am the therapist. It is one of the most difficult transitions I have to make each Friday when I see Dr. Adena at eight in the morning in her suburban office, then make the drive down to the city to arrive at my own office at ten. One Tuesday after the previous Friday's session, she told me she had come into the bathroom and heard me retching into the toilet because the session was so emotional.

On occasion, I feel as though Dr. Adena knows what is on my mind before I have the courage to say it to her; that has proven to be true over the course of the years I have been seeing her. I have a tendency to censor myself. I call it thinking before I speak, but that is merely a form of rationalization. Dr.

Adena is constantly encouraging me, no, pushing me hard to be spontaneous, to say what "comes to mind"—that is one of her favorite expressions—often I do not because I am embarrassed at the words that get caught in my throat. I have gotten better at it over the course of our work together in the four-plus years that we have been working together but I remember once she asked me if I wanted to lie down on the couch, which would have meant not seeing her face. The response was immediate and emphatic. "No."

I have expressed to her that if I were to say whatever comes to my mind without thinking about it, the result would be a psychotic string of unconnected words that would make no sense. That is known as 'word salad' and is typical of those diagnosed with schizophrenia. Dr. Adena has told me patiently and repeatedly that this is impossible because I do not have a thought disorder, but I remain skeptical. When my multiple depressions were most severe, they came with the psychotic symptoms of auditory hallucinations, or hearing voices. It was terrifying and to this day I remember the chant that then made sense, but now seems like nonsense and that permeated my very sick brain.

Dr. Adena was the first therapist with whom I was ever able to discuss sex, use the correct terms for vagina, clitoris, and penis—and this seemingly simple feat took approximately three years into our work. She was the first therapist with whom I was ever able to discuss masturbation. I saw my prior therapist for thirteen years and the general subject of sex, much less specifics, never came up. I asked Dr. Adena what she thought the reason was and she said one would be surprised how many therapists there are who are afraid to discuss the issue of sex in their practice.

At the four-year point in our work, I felt Dr. Adena suspected I was having erotic fantasies that involved her and me; I just refused to acknowledge and discuss them out of shame and humiliation. Additionally, there was a fear that once I verbalized them they would hang exposed in the air and I would neither be able to deny them nor take them back. I was also afraid that Dr. Adena would reject me out of disgust and my extreme display of neediness for her. Intellectually, I knew she had most likely seen it all before in her twenty-plus years as an analyst. But that didn't make it any easier for me.

My neediness came out in other ways since I was unable to directly express it to her. I began having 'accidents' which Dr. Adena believes were driven by my unconscious—my way of getting care from medical professionals other than her. At one point last fall, I made so many trips to the emergency room and was actually admitted to the hospital twice, that Dr. Adena told me she had consulted with other clinicians and informed me that if this "acting-out" behavior continues, she will end treatment with me. Additionally, I missed so much work due to the hospitalizations, and leaving work early/ coming in late due to doctor's appointments, that Ellen sat me down and asked me if a full-time job was too stressful for me.

During that same period, Dr. Adena asked me if I would like to increase our sessions from two to three times a week to try to cope with the intense feelings and acting-out behaviors in which the erotic transference was resulting. I agreed, knowing that it would use up all my savings and that I could not tell any of my friends or family; they already thought Dr. Adena was exploiting me by seeing me twice a week for more than four years.

It took seven months of three-times-per-week sessions of intense work that left me feeling drained, anxious and terrified as I walked out of Dr. Adena's office. I often left in tears and stopped in the bathroom to collect myself. Dr. Adena keeps strict analytic boundaries—she is not one to extend the session past forty-five minutes even if one is sobbing.

All I recall about that particular session is that it was a Friday morning—then I had to leave her office and go to work. I remember driving down to the city afterwards, the session running like a slow-motion horror film in my mind. I was very distracted and I couldn't stay in my lane. I was lucky I didn't have an accident and if there had been a police car near me, he would have likely pulled me over for drunk driving.

It began with an admission that yes, I had been, for some time developing an erotic fantasy in which the two of us, Dr. Adena and I, had been engaging in sex. I described it to her in tears, shaking, my voice cracking, hesitating at times, forcing myself to go on increasing in detail, with gentle encouraging questions from her. I could not meet her eyes, I was so humiliated. When I was finally done, I looked at her and apologized, "I'm sorry." I choked out.

"Why are you apologizing?" She sounded genuinely surprised.

I don't remember what I said. It was probably something to do with involving her in this disgusting, dirty, perverted fantasy.

All day at work I kept picturing the two of us together as I had described it to her in the fantasy. It popped up during the most inappropriate times—when I was in session with a patient, when I was in my supervisor's office. I couldn't wait to leave. Saturday was worse. I woke up from a disturbed sleep very early, and called Dr. Adena attempting to leave an emergency message on her voicemail. It wasn't her usual message—her voicemail was out of order. I wasn't suicidal but I was having self-destructive urges. I didn't know if she would be angry with me for doing this, but I called the psychiatrist who covers for her when she is on vacation and asked her to get in touch with Dr. Adena via her cell phone. Finally, later that afternoon, my phone rang.

I was crying and she had a difficult time understanding me.

"I can't take this." I said. "I'm going crazy. I shouldn't have told you. It was a mistake. I wish I could take it back."

"It wasn't a mistake." she assured me. "You're not going crazy."

I remember her asking me if I was safe. "I don't know," I wailed.

"If you feel like you're going to hurt yourself, then you have to go to the ER," she directed me.

As the sessions ran into each other following this monumental one, my love for Dr. Adena grew, both erotically, and in my feeling of admiration for her intelligence and skill. The realization ensued that I desperately needed her to optimize the other aspects of my life. Her interpretation was that I have to work through this erotic transference in order to be able to achieve successful intimate relationships with men—something that I have not yet been able to do either emotionally or sexually.

One of the understood goals of erotic transference is to finally understand the profound difference between 'desire' and 'love'—something that escapes me in the therapeutic sense. Then having worked through one's defenses, one's intense desire for a single person, one can proceed to offer genuine 'love' to everyone.

My premise to her is that I live in terror of what horrors my brain is capable of continuing to manufacture. Adding to my fear, I am afraid that my erotic love and subsequent fantasies for her will drive me over the edge—again. It has happened before; I have become psychotic but I have come back; only this time I will not come back from the insanity. Even Dr. Adena, with all her skill and expertise, will not be able to bring me back from that dark world, plagued by the voices.

Dancing that fine line, balancing on the edge of that cliff where in my mind insanity awaits despite Dr. Adena's reassurance that it is impossible, terrorizes me during sessions with her and outside of the safety of her office. She continues to push me to go forward, to speak what "comes to mind" without censoring my most intimate thoughts.

"I can't, I won't." My body reacts. I feel nauseous. Like I am going to retch. And I remember that fateful weekend.

Although that weekend has passed and my body has survived intact, I feel my psyche was scarred; my perception of myself was altered as I have now labeled myself as terribly perverted.

Love and insanity. It is a fine line. It's a tightrope I walk every time I enter Dr. Adena's office aware that my purpose is to strip my psyche down to its core. Will the intensity of my love for her drive me to lose my precarious balance so I slip off that narrow rope into the abyss of insanity? Every session is a question mark. And so far, I remain sane.

I find myself teetering dangerously on that rope when I allow this forbidden thought to occasionally leak from my unconscious—that transferential love is not mutual. There is no love towards me on the part of Dr. Adena except perhaps in my fantasies. I would have to be delusional to truly believe that my love for my analyst is being returned with even one millimeter of the intensity for which I care for her. Her concern for me remains strictly on a professional level.

In order to regain my footing I have been forced to seek out, to create for myself other passions to sustain me between my sessions over the long and empty weekends. Patients with borderline personality disorder typically have great difficulty with a concept known as "object constancy," an example of which is when a person whom the patient cares about leaves or is separated from her (even temporarily). Then the patient may have a problem recreating or remembering feelings of love or affection that were present between them when they were physically together.

What sustains me, primarily on the weekends when I head to my local café with my laptop, is my passion for writing. It fulfills me, it nourishes my psyche, my spirit and my soul, taking me places that I did not know existed. Ironically I started writing the essay that would become my first published memoir about my struggle with anorexia while I was an inpatient on an eating disorder unit: the one where I was so angry with Dr. Adena for hospitalizing me when I believed she reneged on our contract. Being separated from her for an extended period of time forced me to find an alternate method of coping with the pain of longing and desire for her. For some reason, the act of putting pen to paper, finding that rhythm, that flow of writing, connecting the words, soothed me in a way that nothing else could.

I see writing as creating something from nothing; where a blank tablet existed just minutes prior, I have left my mark with a unique combination of words, sentences, paragraphs that meld into a larger form. It is a message from me to my readers, where I opt to be brutally honest about the intimate, inner workings of my conscious mind (and a smattering of my unconscious); otherwise, it seems to me that the message falls short and the reader will sense that I am holding back.

It feels as if the power of words, the power of my words communicating what has been the insanity of my life, makes me increasingly sane. The more I write, the more I expose, serves to demystify the stigma of the "craziness" for the layman. And when those close to me tell me they cannot read what I have written for it hurts them too much to know what I have endured all these years—then I know I have succeeded.

When I write, I lose myself. Do I dare say it's the only time I don't feel ill? Ironically, I write about the dark world I used to inhabit on a daily basis, the destructive acts I used to perpetrate on myself in such a variety of creative, innovative ways and how much I wanted to die, but I am able to contain those feelings to the paper. When I go back to a piece after I have been separated from it for some time, after it has gone through the publishing process and the copies have arrived in a cardboard box (my essays printed along with the essays of others of a similar theme), I read it and those of the other contributors and then I gaze at the printed words, half in horror, and half in awe. Did I really do those things to myself? Was I really capable of that? Was I really so ill? And then I want to throw up.

I often think when I write how much I must have hated and loathed myself to be able to do those things to my body and my spirit, but once I write them down and share them, they lose their power to be so horrific. Incidents that once caused me to put in emergency calls to Dr. Adena on weekend afternoons no longer leave me curled up quivering in a fetal position awaiting her return phone call. Written down, fragments of thoughts that fail to make sense turn into coherent sentences and then I have an entire essay and my sanity has returned.

Not just writing, but the art of what I perceive as intimate, open, honest writing, not to shock but with the intention of allowing the reader into an inner sanctum, is critical to maintaining my balance on that tightrope where insanity awaits in the abyss below and sanity is at the other end of the platform. There is the admittedly tortuous process of writing to meet deadlines, submissions, waiting anxiously for a response, revisions and more revisions if accepted, or rejections more often than not. During this process I precariously blow in the wind on that tightrope. It is extremely difficult to endure but it is part of being a writer. I cannot starve myself to deal with the pain of a rejection because a brain that lacks proper nutrition cannot function to write coherently and I want to continue writing more than I want to be a size 00. But, the thought still persists because I have been anorexic for twenty-three years and the hold of the disease does not let go that easily. I know that I will always fight that stubborn urge.

Just as I came to writing later in life, I also made the decision to return to graduate school to obtain my masters in social work and become a therapist. During all my psychotherapy, as ill as I was, I became fascinated by the process: "How did the therapist know what to say to me, what questions to ask during the session?" I would walk away from the therapy hour thinking these things to myself and when I was capable I would read books on the therapeutic process.

I soon came to the conclusion that psychotherapy is more of an art than a science. There is no course in graduate school entitled, "How to Conduct A Therapy Session," although there probably should be. The back-and-forth of my first session was akin to initially driving on a highway after receiving a learner's permit. So many things to pay attention to—facial expressions, body gestures, tone of voice—while trying to focus on the road ahead: the patient.

My first counseling session was conducted while completing my internship during my second year of graduate school. It was with a young woman who was diagnosed with depression, borderline personality disorder, and anorexia (it was like looking into a mirror). My assignment was to try to get her to drink an Ensure (Ensures are high calorie liquid nutritional supplements that are often given as an addition to food when a patient needs to gain weight.) Of course I did not succeed and I felt as if I were an incompetent failure. I was able to empathize with her because she was me or I was her and maybe that got in the way.

I use my work with my patients to recognize problems within myself, promote my own personal growth and most importantly continually work on becoming a better therapist. When my patients express an interest in entering the field of social work, as I did when I was in therapy, I am honest with them and tell them it is extremely rewarding work that requires a great deal of patience, for a course of therapy often takes years, but at the same time it is not a nine-to-five job. I think about and I am concerned for my patients as I drive home from the office, when I am stuck in traffic, as I stand in line at Dunkin' Donuts for my coffee and bagel on a weekend morning. I am incapable of cutting off my concern for them when I leave the office at the end of the day

The blaring problem within me that resonates in my work with patients is neediness. I've talked about how much I need Dr. Adena, and naturally my patients have come to need me on a regular basis, they have come to look forward to seeing me weekly or twice-weekly depending on their individual schedule. They get angry when I am out sick, or I take a personal day or a week of vacation, as if I do not have the right—and they demand to be seen at another time. If they have to cancel, they expect that I will be able to squeeze them into my schedule at another time during the week as if I do not have other patients to consider. This is an example of their lack of object constancy. They are unable to carry a sense of me through until their next session, especially if they miss their weekly appointment and the gap stretches into two weeks.

Many of my patients have great difficulty keeping to the limits of the forty-five minute session. When I point out that it is time to stop for the day, they continue to talk as if they haven't heard me. I repeat myself more firmly, "We really have to end for today." And they sit motionless in their chair. The way the daily schedule is structured at my clinic, the therapists have only five minutes between sessions to use the restroom and/or write the session note and by now those five minutes have been used up and at this point I am feeling angry and resentful. What it comes down to is reluctance on the part of the patients to separate from someone who might be the one person in their life by whom they feel listened, understood, and not judged.

I usually address this issue with the patients by talking about the concept of respect for the patient following them. I point out that they are causing me to be late for the next patient and they would not like it if I was late coming out to get them from the waiting room and their session was shortened. They are usually capable of understanding that line of reasoning. They may get angry, accusing me of "cutting them off," but then I suggest they use their time between sessions to think about what we were discussing and to come back next session ready to explore it in greater depth.

The major difference between being seen in a clinic such as the one in which I work that accepts various forms of insurance and often, Medicaid and Medicare, and seeing a therapist or psychiatrist in private practice who does not accept insurance, is that when one misses a session with the latter regardless of the reason, one still is required to pay the full fee. When a patient cancels at a clinic, there is no such requirement. I've had patients cancel, beg to be rescheduled and then just not show up for the rescheduled appointment without even calling.

This particular behavior brings up a range of feelings within me as the therapist. The fact that they practically demand/expect to be seen after canceling with no consequences, makes me feel like a mere convenience, a cast-off but then when they do request to be rescheduled I feel like they do value their time with me and believe that they can benefit from a session.

Their demanding, entitled expectations as if they are the only patient on my schedule is a defense against a certain level of neediness and dependence, which irritates me and makes me angry though I cannot express that to them. All I can say to them is that I have no openings at the moment but if a cancellation comes up, I will give them a call. I say that to them in such a way that allows them to realize that I have other patients on my schedule and then they have no other choice but to accept that.

This both subtle and overt neediness reminds me of the desperate dependence I feel towards Dr. Adena that I am working so hard to overcome. When I describe such a scenario to her she notes from my tone of voice (and I don't even realize this is how I am coming across) that I get punitive in my attitude towards a patient who displays such behavior towards me. My feelings of neediness for Dr. Adena spill over into my countertransference towards my patients. I loathe myself for being so needy, so dependent, and I cannot seem to tolerate the fact that anyone would feel the same way with a similar intensity toward me.

I sometimes feel that I can't handle what I can experience as my clients' intense need of me, their therapist. As I gain more insight into my own neediness, I sometimes say, "Maybe I am in the wrong profession." But that is a fleeting thought. The feedback I get from some of my patients

("You've helped me so much.") nourishes and validates me in the same way receiving an acceptance letter from a publisher does.

Regardless of this back-and-forth inner dialogue, I love my job. I look forward to going into the office each morning. The ten, eleven-hour day goes by very quickly. Along with writing, it is truly a calling, a passion. It sustains me during the week between sessions. When I first went back to work after a two-year absence, I had no confidence in my abilities and I kept comparing myself to Dr. Adena, who obviously has had much more training and experience than I have had. I kept a running dialogue in my head during a session with a patient: "Is this what Dr. Adena would say?" Now I no longer feel the need to play this internal tape because my confidence in my skills has grown exponentially.

I give of myself to my patients and they give much more of themselves to me. They lay out their bare, naked, honest truths to me and look at me expectantly as if I know the answer that will end their suffering. I realize that even after all these years I have the same expectations of Dr. Adena. My love for her blinds me to her 'humanness' and her faults. Sometimes in my own practice, I do know what to say and it comes forward rather readily. Often I do not know what to say so I stay silent and listen and ask seemingly pertinent questions. Often I am afraid of asking questions that will probe and hurt or giving feedback that will provoke anger even though I know one of several possible correct interpretations.

I know this from my own life, from my own years and years as a patient in therapy and from what I endure while I am outside the therapy office where I work so hard with Dr. Adena. My psyche remains a dangerous place, a conglomeration of treatment from both superior and incompetent therapists, from acts of self-destruction to positive steps of self-affirmation— like writing and working as a therapist. My gut experiences something different because it is prenatal, preverbal; it twists and turns, often fighting my mind for what it wants, because it desires primitive, destructive forms of self-soothing. The almost constant conflict creates a war which rages inside my body; the anxiety escalates and it comes back to an agonizing choice between regressing back to the safety of my long-time illness or reflecting on my accomplishments and moving forward to what I am potentially capable of as a writer and a psychotherapist. The terror, the conflict is indescribable.

There remains within me a very fine line between love and insanity. I walk the line each day, each hour. Some days I am able to sustain myself primarily through the writer within me, the therapist within me; other days I need to hear more of Dr. Adena's wise words, to drink in the fine features of her face. There are days when my hold on my sense of sanity is more tenuous than others. I know I am resilient because I want to live and work and write although sometimes it hurts so badly. Love is a feeling; passion for writing is a feeling. Insanity is not a feeling; it is just a state of existence and right now in my life I want more to feel even if it hurts then to merely exist. That is more sane than insane.

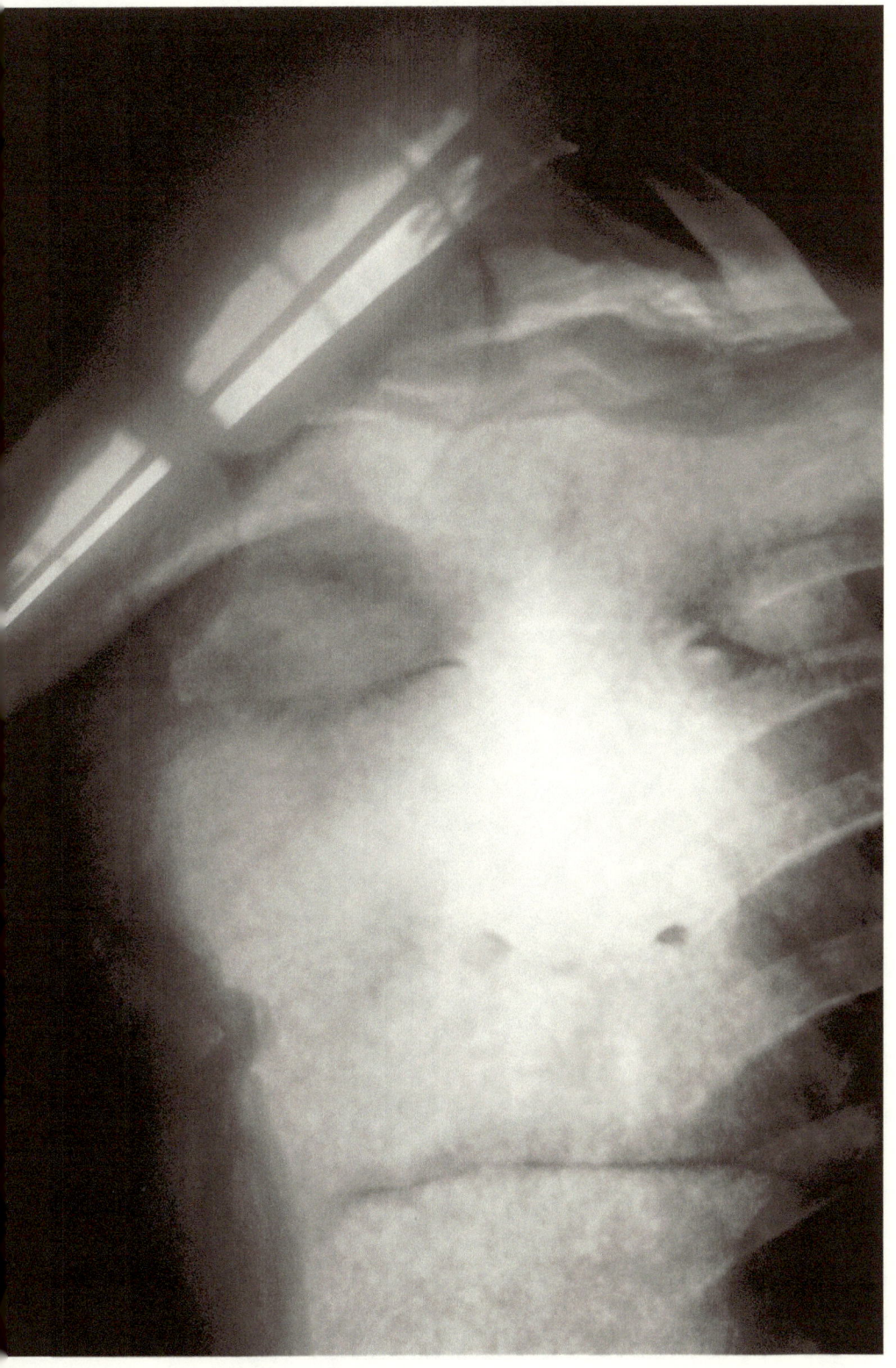

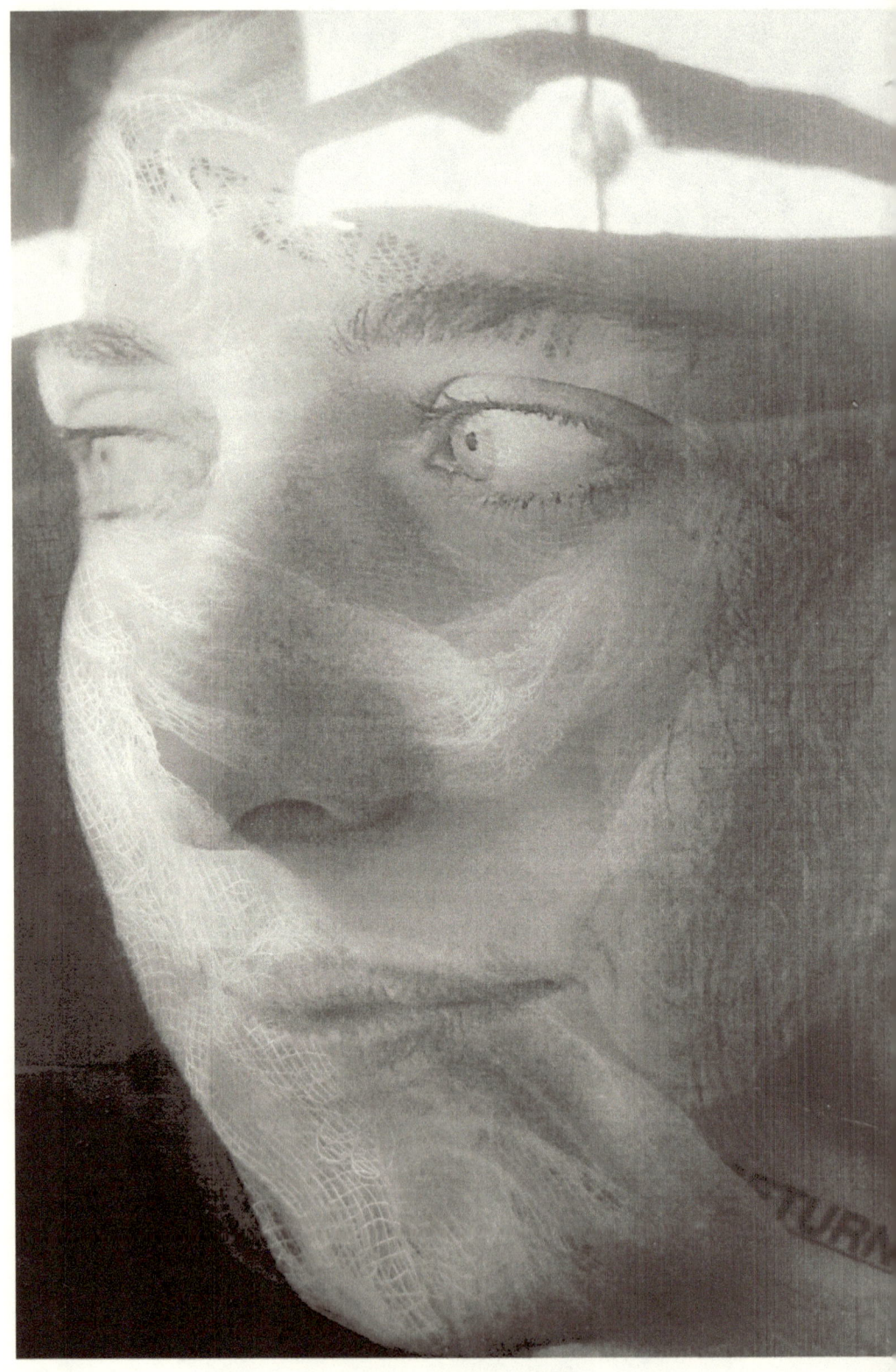

DISCUSSION GUIDE

I. IMMEDIATE EXPERIENCE

In a number of the poems in this section, one has the sense of someone pausing in a doorway, startled into seeing anew. In some ways that positioning is echoed by us as readers, pausing to turn the page, to enter into yet another sensibility, pivotal, aware of the power of our gaze. Sometimes we need to return again to beginner's mind in order to see straight and fresh. There is so much talk about medicine, about sickness, about health, with or without the care. But what gets us is the real stuff—the loopy paean we want to sing to our anesthesiologist as we go under, the combination of the ordinary and the mysterious in a technician's dance that shocks us out of our tragic stance, the unapologetically bared breasts of a dying woman and the faint citrus mist we add to the situation.

1) What particular images in these selections catch in your imagination? Are there images from your own experiences, bed or bedside, that keep coming back to you and asking to be explored?

2) The narrator in "Clay" finds the bared breasts of Grace, her dying patient, disorienting. She seems to be searching for a distance that is both empathic and professionally detached and that allows her to meet Grace exactly where she is. Who do you see as the wiser of the two? What is the most valuable thing that each woman offers to the other?

3) Molly O'Dell's poems combine a poet's eye and a physician's distance. As a reader, do you have a desire to know more, come closer or do these vivid snapshots feel complete to you? Why?

4) Why do you think the therapist in Sylvie Terespolski's story finds his patient so challenging? Who feels more reality-based to you?

II. BOUNDARIES

Roles, professional and personal, are defined as much by what we won't do as by what we will. Professions define themselves by drawing an essential line between the members within its charmed sphere and those outside it. That line is both comforting, since it defines expert knowledge, but is also problematic when the emphasis is not on medical knowledge but care, which regularly brings us, sick and well, into skin contact with one another. What boundaries apply then? How permeable do these boundaries need to be if care is to be expressed and received? Nurses are especially alert to this semi-permeable membrane, the choices involved for them when rigid compliance will cause harm and complete disregard may do the same, when to ignore what a patient has to teach will diminish the world for both of them. As Paula Sergi writes, "Once in awhile/ I'd see it when I washed their bony backs,/ a used-up body about to lift off/on scapular wings."

1) In Kathleen Kelley's "We Go A Little Over the Hour," she writes, "People ask how I bear/listening to endless sorrow./All I can say: it makes a difference." What difference is made in these poems and stories when the nurse or therapist chooses to meet their patient at the patient's boundary rather than insisting the patient meet them at their own customary one?

2) Sometimes people are not comforted by words. Reflect back on a time when the most comfort you could share was your presence. How did you show compassion without using words, or violating physical or emotional boundaries?

3) What different boundaries, professional and personal, do the narrators in Rachel Bloom's poems chafe at?

4) In Phyllis Langton's "Dying at Home," what boundaries does she respect? Which ones does she challenge? What helps her draw her lines?

III. LONG-TERM RELATIONSHIPS

Long-term relationships are, by their very nature, complex, messy with history and shifting needs. They also ask something more and different from physician and patient, something each party might be just as happy to do without if they could. But could that extra something enrich all doctor-patient relations, however brief? How would you define the shifting relationship to health and wholeness that takes place when diseases are accepted as chronic and, possibly, as Timothy Urban realizes, fundamentals of the human condition?

1) Nancy Brandwein in her memoir "My Doctor and I" describes her long-term relationship with her doctor as like a marriage—and also immediately identifies how it differs from a marriage because of the inequality of information and power of the participants. What simile or metaphor would you use to describe her long-term relationship with her doctor? What does she want from him? What do you think it is realistic for her to expect?

2) In Evelyn Sharenov's memoir, "Annie," Annie accuses her of being neutral, but the narrator says, "When I thought of Annie I felt weary and sad. I wanted to grab her by the shoulders and shake some sense into her; definitely not neutral." Reading this account of a difficult, intense, long-term relationship, do *you* feel neutral? If not, what emotions do you feel?

3) In "Davin's Angel," what begins to change in Zoë Losada's relationship with the doctors and nurses who are caring for her son? When does this change take place? Is it when she gives up hope of a permanent solution—or when they experience, at long last, a 'successful' outcome?

4) How does Timothy Urban's relationship with his existential therapist differ from Brandwein's relationship with her internist? Why?

IV. DEFINING EXPERIENCE: THE POWER OF WORDS

"I still can't get my head around/ other people's pain being any/ different from mine," writes Paul Hostovsky in his poem "Other People's Pain." But even his ability to understand this cornerstone of empathy is compromised by how his dentist responded, defined, his own experience of pain at the age of ten. In all the selections in this section, people are defining, intentionally or not, the subjective experience of others in ways that can either increase or relieve their pain. What makes the difference?

1) In Matthew Smith's "The Gift," what makes him open to the quiet remonstrance of his patient? What was she criticizing exactly? Do you think most physicians you have met would respond similarly if you noted how their word choice, quality of attention, or use of time affected your experience of care?

2) In Mariette Landry's "Talking" and Claudia Van Gerven's "As Benign as Breast Tissue Can Be," the conversation of their doctors is experienced as worse than indifferent. Have you had similar experiences? Do you think saying anything would have changed things?

3) In many of these stories about pregnancy and childbirth, the responses of nurses strongly influence how the women experience their condition, especially their sense of responsibility and their own agency. Do you think the nurses are aware of the amount of influence they have to define this experience for women? Why is the power to define greater here than if the women were having a broken leg set or high blood pressure treated?

V. ERRORS

"A Himalayan ice crevasse is smaller than the emotional distance surgeons must leap in a heartbeat between empathy and focused indifference. The risks are deadly if you miss your footing," writes David Page in "Burr Holes in the Heart." There is also the distance patients must cross when they live out the consequences of medical error—which is not the same as malfeasance, although our leg may be split just as wide, our cornea be as deeply scarred, our lungs and legs as dangerously filled with fluid. Does the 'why' matter? Crucially, it seems. As does the ability to acknowledge fallibility. But does error or bad outcome require apology and forgiveness? Does the fallibility of our doctor require of us a state of sustained vigilance in the future?

1) Jane Herschlag's poems move back and forth between early trauma and medical incompetence or oversight. How responsible is the physician treating the current problem for the troubling and potentially traumatizing intersection of these two powerful experiences, past and present? Are they the source of poetry rather than malpractice suits?

2) The memoirs and stories in this section that take the patient's point of view usually reflect something the patient was not allowed to say or do inside the situation—and so can be read as an attempt to repair their own helplessness. Are there experiences you have had with healthcare practioners that you have needed to revisit, find words to speak back with, unlearn your helplessness?

3) What makes Diane Payne's story both horrifying and funny?

4) Having read his memoir, would you want to be a patient of David Page? Why or why not?

5) Rita Charon writes in *Narrative Medicine*, "The emotions of shame, blame and fear erect the most unbreachable divides between doctors and patients." Where in the selections in this section do you see these emotions at work? What are their consequences? What bridges need to be built into our healthcare system, as well as between individuals, to span these divides?

VI. GROWING IN OUR ROLES

A role is our function in a particular social situation: mother-child, judge-defense attorney, doctor-patient. Professional competence derives from how well we are able as individuals to fulfill the requirements of that function, but social trust also derives from how well that professional function fits our society's needs. Both these, professional standards and social and systems trust, change over time for reasons that have little to do with individuals—but are experienced most personally all the same. What does it mean to grow in our roles? Does it mean accepting how the system works? Does it mean questioning how well the function fits the situation? Does it mean identifying—or disidentifying? Does it involve developing a hierarchy of roles that counterbalance and thus redefine each other, as Robert Kus observes in the life of Rich Murray?

1) Elaine Morgan in her wry essay, "The Zen and the Art of Medical Appointments," shows us how to play the system. Joel Peckham opts out, deciding he would rather live with chronic pain than keep playing the role of patient. In what situations would you make choices similar to the ones Morgan makes? Are there any situations in which you would choose Peckham's course? Why?

2) Robert Sticca's memoir captures the drama of professionalization, of meeting, or exceeding, the rigorous standards of his profession. What do you think might have happened to this narrator, and to his understanding of himself as a surgeon, if the patient had not made it?

3) Burnout is one of the themes of Nina Gaby's "The Inventories We Keep"— but there is something darker than burnout we glimpse in Claudette Mork Sigg's "The Darkness in Sister Mercy." What is it?

VII. CHANGING PLACES

We will all, whether we want to or not, end up at one time or another taking the view from the bed. John Rawls argues that the only just social systems are the ones where we would be willing to inhabit any role in it. To what extent is healthcare a social system and to what extent does this definition of justice apply? How many of us wish to inhabit the role of patient, the one defined by our ability to bear suffering? And how many of us are willing to let someone who has endured suffering, especially mental suffering, fully recover, to take once and for all another role, become one of us?

1) Several of the selections here—Sharenov, Gaby, and Luce—explore the shifting border between mental illness and mental health. Why is this kind of exploration more likely—and more disturbing—than a surgeon operating after his own surgery, or a nurse receiving nursing care?

2) What has to shift in the narrator of Paula Sergi's story "Survey" for her to be able to acknowledge her own illness? What shifts in Sanville's narrator when he understands his fellow patient to be a doctor? How does the tone in both these stories, which is light, ironic, affect how we respond to these inversions?

3) At some point, most practicing health professionals are also patients. Consequently, they know the experience of losing some autonomy over their behavior and recovery. Is it likely that these experiences will contribute to empathy and understanding that health professionals show their patients so that they able to build healthy relationships?

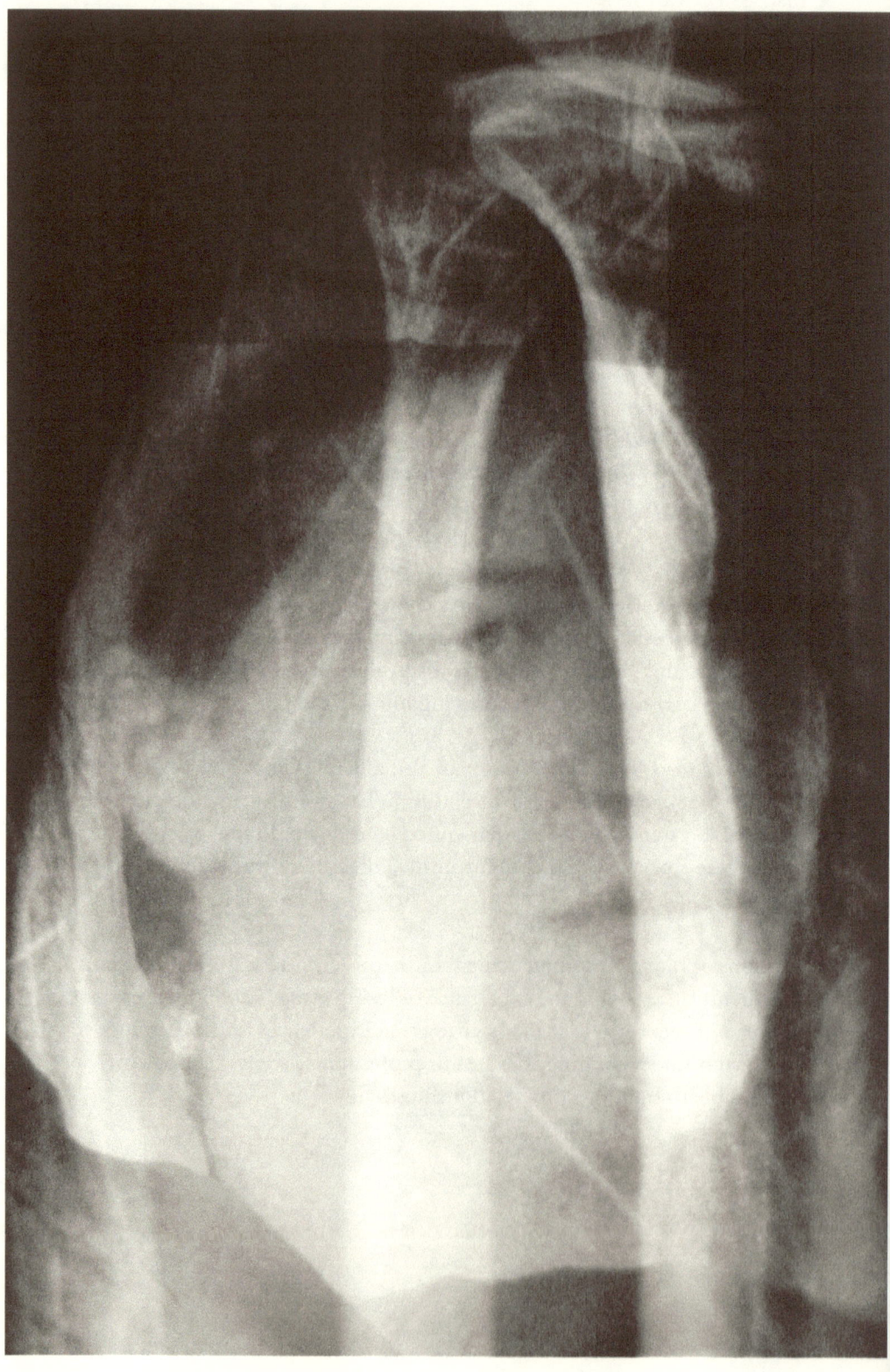

SELECT BIBLIOGRAPHY

John Abramson. *Overdosed America: The Broken Promise of American Medicine.* NY: HarperCollins, 2004.

Kristin Baird. *Reclaiming the Passion: Stories that Celebrate the Essence of Nursing.* Fort Atkinson, WI: Golden Lamp Press, 2004.

Boston Women's Health Collective and Judy Norsigian. *Our Bodies, Ourselves: A New Edition for a New Era.* New York: Touchstone, 2005.

Alida Brill and Michael D. Lockshin. *Dancing at the River's Edge: A Patient and Her Doctor Negotiate Life with Chronic Illness.* Tucson: Schaffner Press, 2009.

Jerome Bruner. *Actual Minds, Possible Worlds.* Cambridge: Harvard University Press, 1986.

_____. *Acts of Meaning.* Cambridge: Harvard University Press, 1990.

Carol Wiley Cassella. *Oxygen.* New York: Simon & Schuster, 2008.

Rita Charon. *Narrative Medicine: Honoring the Stories of Illness.* New York: Oxford University Press, 2006.

Pauline W. Chen. *Final Exam: A Surgeon's Reflections on Mortality.* New York: Alfred A. Knopf, 2007.

_____(Editor). *The Best American Medical Writing.* New York: Kaplan Publishing, 2009.

John L. Coulehan and Marian L. Block. *The Medical Interview: Mastering Skills for Clinical Practice.* Philadelphia: F.A. Davis, 2006.

Norbert Elias. *The Loneliness of the Dying.* New York: Continuum, 2001.

Katrina Firlik. *Another Day in the Frontal Lobe: A Brain Surgeon Exposes Life on the Inside.* New York: Random House, 2006.

Daniel Goleman. *Social Intelligence.* New York: Bantam Books, 2006.

Jerome E. Groopman. *How Doctors Think.* New York: Houghton Mifflin, 2007.

_____. *The Anatomy of Hope: How People Prevail in the Face of Illness.* New York: Random House, 2004.

Thomas Graboys and Peter Zheutlin. *Life in the Balance: A Physician's Memoir of Life, Love and Loss with Parkinson's Disease and Dementia.* New York: Union Square Press, 2008.

David Hilfiker. *Healing the Wounds: A Physician Looks at His Work*. 2nd.
 Rev. ed. Omaha: Creighton University Press, 1998.

Anne Katherine. *Boundaries: Where You End and I Begin*. New York: Simon
 & Schuster, 1991.

Susan Kuner, Carol Osborn, Linda Quigley and Karen Stroup. *Speak the
 Language of Healing: Living With Breast Cancer Without Going to War*.
 Berkeley: Conari Press, 1999.

Vincent Lam, *Bloodletting & Miraculous Cures*. Reprint Edition. New York:
 Weinstein Books, 2008.

George D. Lundberg, M.D. *Severed Trust: Why American Medicine Hasn't
 Been Fixed*. NY: Basic Books, 2000.

Timothy B. McCall. *Examining Your Doctor: A Patient's Guide to Avoiding
 Harmful Medical Care*. New York: Birch Lane Press, 1995.

Dennis McCullough. *My Mother, Your Mother*. NY: HarperCollins, 2008.

Nancy Mairs. *Remembering Bone House*. Boston: Beacon Press, 1995.

Cheryl Mattingly. *Healing Dramas and Clinical Plots: The Narrative Structure
 of Experience*. New York: Cambridge University Press, 2001.

Christina Middlebrook. *Seeing the Crab: A Memoir of Dying*. New York:
 Basic Books, 1996.

Paul Monette. *Borrowed Time: An AIDS Memoir*. New York: Mariner Books,
 2008.

Ruth Nadelhaft (Editor) with Victoria Bonnebakker. *Imagine What It's Like:
 A Literature and Medicine Anthology*. University of Hawaii Press, 2008.

Sherwin P. Nuland. *The Soul of Medicine*. NY: Kaplan Publishers, 2009.

Susan Pories, Sachin H. Jain, and Gordon Harper. *The Soul of a Doctor:
 Harvard Medical Students Face Life and Death*. Chapel Hill, NC:
 Algonquin Books, 2006.

Cheri Register. *The Chronic Illness Experience*. Hazelden, Center City,
 Minneapolis, 1987.

Rachel Naomi Remen. *Kitchen Table Wisdom: Stories that Heal*. New York:
 Riverhead Books, 1997.

____. *My Grandfather's Blessings: Stories of Strength, Refuge and Belonging*.
 New York: Riverhead Books, 2000.

Lisa Sanders. *Every Patient Tells a Story*. NY: Broadway Books, 2009.

Matthew Sanford. *Waking: A Memoir of Trauma and Transcendence*.
 Minneapolis: Rodale Books, 2008.

Lisa Kennedy Sheldon. *Communication for Nurses: Talking with Patients.* Sudbury, MA: Jones and Bartlett Publishers, 2009.

Amy Silverstein. *Sick Girl.* New York: Grove Press, 2007.

John Tarrant. *The Light Inside the Dark.* New York: HarperPerennial, 1998.

Jill Bolte Taylor. *My Stroke of Insight: A Brain Scientist's Personal Journey.* New York: Viking, 2008.

Emily R. Transue. *Patient by Patient.* NY: St. Martin's Press, 2008.

Abraham Verghese. *My Own Country: A Doctor's Story.* New York: Vintage, 1995.

Marilyn Walton. *The Trouble with Medicine: Preserving the Trust Between Patients and Doctors.* Allen & Unwin Academic, 1999.

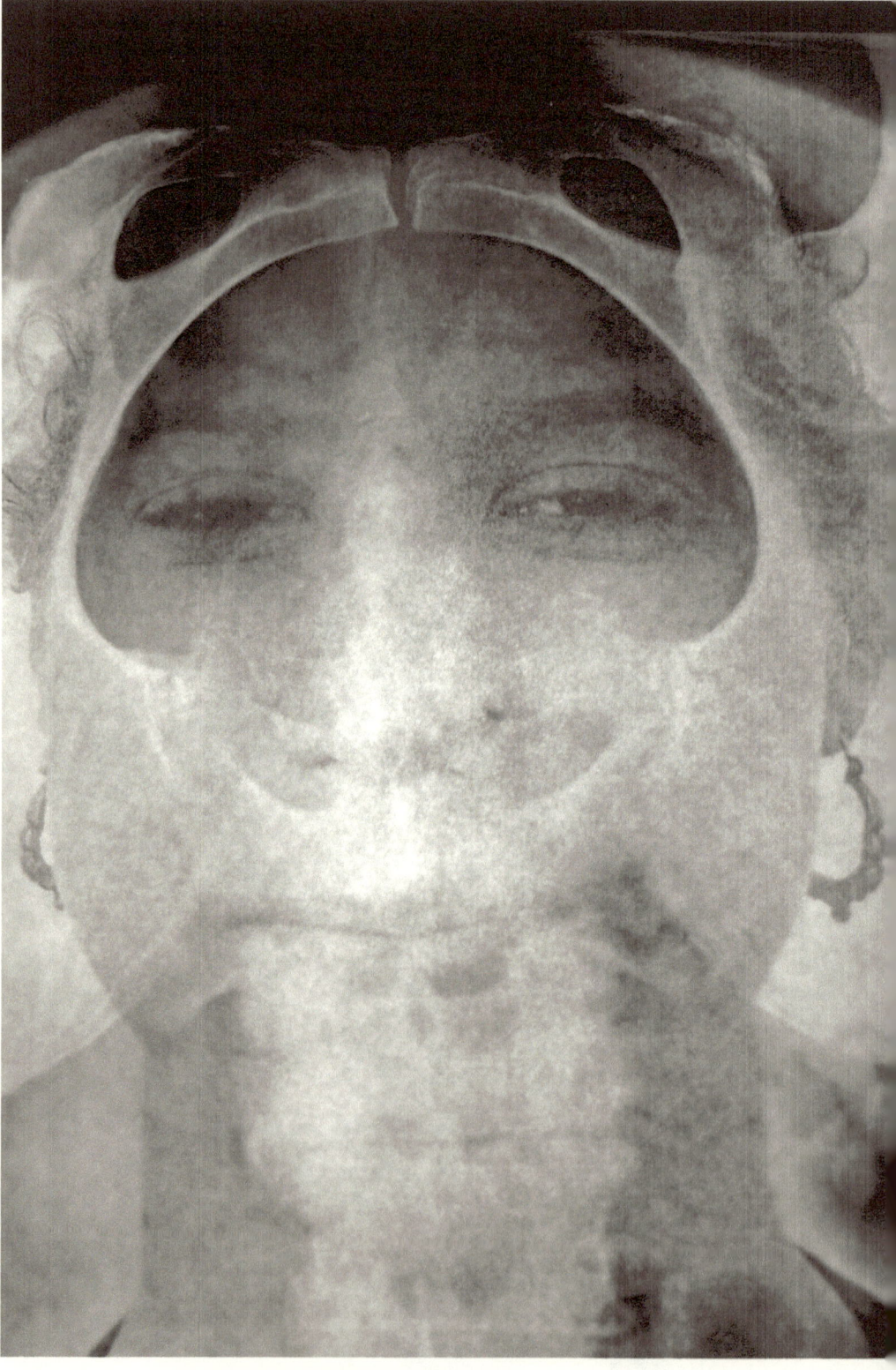

ACKNOWLEDGEMENTS

Paul Hostovsky's "Psalm," "Other People's Pain," and "The Nurse's Office" are reprinted from his *Dear Truth* (Main Street Rag, 2009).

Kathleen M. Kelley published "We Go a Little Over the Hour" and "If I Could Paint Them" in the chapbook *The Waiting Room* (Providence Athenaeum, 2010); the former also appeared in slightly different form in *Women's Encounters with the Mental Health Establishment: Escaping the Yellow Wallpaper*, ed. Elayne Clift (Haworth Press, 2002).

Mariette Landry's "Freedom Trail" was previously published in *New Voices Anniversary Edition* (Heatherstone Press, 1992).

Sara Lippmann's "Girl" was previously published in *All Things Girl* (www.allthingsgirl.net).

John Manesis's "Wen" is reprinted from his *With All My Breath* (Cosmos Publishing Co.).

Paula Sergi's "Home Visits" was previously published in *Intensive Care: More Poetry & Prose by Nurses* (University of Iowa Press and *The Sow's Ear Poetry Review*) and "Sudden Wrinkle" in *American Journal of Nursing* (2004).

Evelyn Sharenov's "Annie" was first published in *Etude* (Winter 2008) and "Collateral Damage" in *Citadel of the Spirit* (2009).

Gary Young's "The Tumor Is Small" originally appeared in *Quick Fiction* (number 11).

Photographs by Heather Tosteson, who thanks all those who generously donated an image of their face—or bones—for art. Special thanks to all the members of Atlanta Family Healthcare who graciously did so on a busy day.

We thank Davin Losada for his careful reading and thoughtful response to the manuscript.

Matthew Bishop provided valuable help in the copy editing, proofing and production of the book.

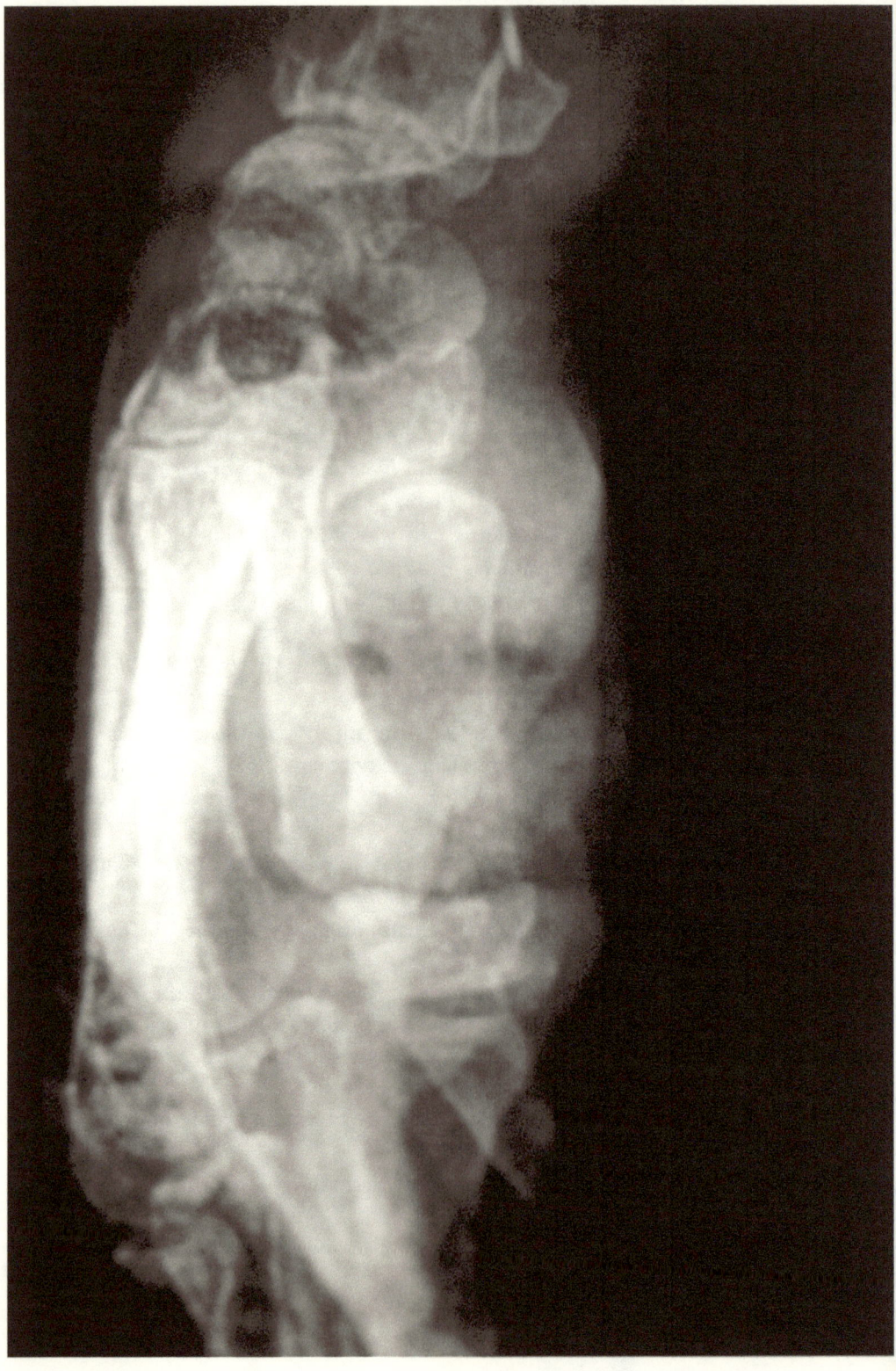

AUTHORS

Patricia Barone has published a book of poetry, *Handmade Paper*, and a novella, *The Wind*, with New Rivers Press. Her poetry and short stories have appeared in anthologies such as *Bless Me Father* (Plume/Penguin) and *One Parish Over: Irish-American Writing* (New Rivers Press); and in periodicals including *New Verse News*, *An Sionnach*, *The Shop*, *Pleiades*, *Commonweal*, *The Seattle Review*, *Visions International*, and *Widener Review*. She has received a Loft-McKnight Award of Distinction in poetry.

Rachel Squires Bloom was born in Boston, Massachusetts. Her poems have appeared in *The Hawaii Review*, *Poet Lore*, *Fugue*, *Poetry East*, *Kimera*, *Nomad's Choir*, *Mad Poet's Review*, *Bluster*, *Bellowing Ark*, *Slugfest*, *Thin Air*, *Taproot Literary Review*, *True Romance*, *Lucid Stone* and *Green Hills Literary Lantern*. She holds Master's degrees in English Literature and in Education, as well as a Doctorate in Educational Leadership. She is a teacher in Quincy, Massachusetts.

Ann J. Brady works as a Symptom Management RN in a Cancer Center. She is currently at work on her MSN. Previous publications include an essay, *I Lied*, which appeared in the September 2009 issue of *Oncology Nursing News*. She is just finishing her first novel.

Nancy J. Brandwein is a freelance writer and probably the only GI tract-challenged food columnist around. Her weekly column, "Snack Attack," appears in the *West Side Spirit*, and she has published essays and feature stories in *The West Side Spirit* as well as in *AM-NY, WHERE-NY, The New York Times* and *Brain, Child*. She lives in New York City with her husband and two children.

Mary Ann DiMola has been a nurse for thiry-two years. Her experience includes burn/critical care nursing, staff/management development, and university teaching. She has many publications related to burn nursing and healthcare education. She earned her M.A. at Teachers College, Columbia University and her Ph.D. at The George Washington University. She is currently a part-time faculty member at The George Washington University and owns a healthcare data business in Bethesda MD.

Nina Gaby is a writer, visual artist, advanced practice nurse and ex-innkeeper living in central Vermont and currently, happily, works as the Clinical Director for a recovery-based residential psychiatric facility. She recently has been published in *Lilith,* and two Seal Press anthologies, and has an essay awaiting publication in *American Funeral Director Magazine.* Her art is included in the National Collection of the Smithsonian as well as other collections, and she runs a studio/gallery. She is, of course, working on a novel.

Jane Herschlag won many poetry awards from Hunter College and City College in New York City. She was a semi-finalist in *Radcliffe's* 2000 Bunting Fellowship, and *Elixir's* 2006 poetry contest. Her poems have appeared in three anthologies: *Queen of Swords, Rising To The Dawn,* and *Writing Our Way Out Of The Dark,* and in many university presses. Her docu-poetry collection, *Bully In The Spotlight,* was published by *Pudding House Publications.*

Paul Hostovsky's poems have won a Pushcart Prize, the Muriel Craft Bailey Award from *The Comstock Review,* and chapbook contests from Grayson Books, Riverstone Press, Frank Cat Press, and Split Oak Press. He has been featured on *Poetry Daily, Verse Daily, The Writer's Almanac,* and *Best of the Net 2008* and *2009.* He has two full-length collections, *Bending the Notes* (2008), and *Dear Truth* (2009).

Kathleen M. Kelley resides in western Massachusetts where she lives in a co-housing community, works as a hospice social worker, spends as much time as possible in nature, and writes poetry, memoir, and essays. Her work has appeared in *Peregrine, The Equinox, The Sun, Many Hands, The Green Fuse, Evergreen Chronicles, Mediphores,* and *Earth's Daughters.* She was the recipient of the 2008 Anderbo Poetry Prize and the 2010 Philbrick Poetry Award.

Patricia Kett is a retired registered nurse for whom writing has been love, work, obsession, play, and escape for over sixty years. While working as a nurse she studied writing and had health related articles and poetry published in local newspapers and books. She is a member of the Upper Delaware Writers Collective in Narrowsburg, NY and has participated in poetry readings in New York, Pennsylvania and New Jersey.

Fr. Robert J. Kus, R.N., Ph.D. is Pastor of St. Mary Catholic Church in Wilmington, NC. Ordained a Catholic priest in 1998, Fr. Bob is also a sociologist, psychiatric-mental health nurse, columnist for Spanish magazines, writer, and university professor. Before becoming a priest, Fr. Bob was an Associate Professor at The University of Iowa. He currently teaches part-time at University of North Carolina at Pembroke.

Mariette Landry has published poetry and short fiction in literary magazines including *Poetry East, Indiana Review, North American Review*, and *Narrative*, and in the anthologies *Microfiction* (Norton) and *Brevity & Echo* (Rose Metal Press). She lives in Boston.

Sara Lippmann writes, lives, and battles the ever-leaky sippy cup in Brooklyn. Her work can be found in the current issue of *Slice Magazine* and is forthcoming from *Fiction Circus* and *Word Riot*.

Zoë Losada was born in Washington, D.C. but has lived more than thirty years in South and Central America, primarily in Venezuela, where she currently makes her home and works as a school counselor. Both her children were born in Venezuela, including her son, Davin, about whom she writes in this anthology.

Gerri Luce, a Licensed Clinical Social Worker, publishes under a pseudonym. Her memoirs explore her experiences with mental illness, anorexia, and healing.

Fredricka R. Maister is a freelance writer who lives in New York City. Her essays and articles have appeared in a variety of publications, including *The Baltimore Sun, Chicago Tribune, The Miami Herald, The Philadelphia Inquirer, Big Apple Parent, New York/Long Island Woman, Coping with Cancer Magazine, Jewish Journal of Greater Los Angeles*, and in the archives of the United States Holocaust Memorial Museum.

John Manesis, born in Eau Claire, Wisconsin in 1936, lives with his wife in Fargo, North Dakota. He is a retired physician whose poetry has appeared in sixty literary publications, including *Charioteer, Measure, North Dakota Quarterly, Wisconsin Review*, and *Lyric*. His first poetry book, *With All My Breath*, was published in 2003 by Cosmos and the second, *Other Candle Lights*, was published by Seaburn Publishing in 2008.

Michele Markarian's plays have been published by Dramatic Publishing and Heuer Publishing, and have been produced throughout the United States and Great Britain. Her short story *Shake* was published in the anthology *Families: The Frontline of Pluralism* (Wising Up Press, 2008). Michele has also written for *Mom's Literary Magazine*, *Regional Air Cargo Review* and *The Air Charter Journal*. Michele is a member of the Dramatists Guild of America.

Carolyn McAuliffe resides in Southern California with her husband Mike and son Michael. She holds a Master of Fine Arts in Creative Writing from San Diego State University. Carolyn's writing resume includes: book editor of an educational textbook published by Greenhaven Press, an adjunct-faculty position teaching English Composition, and currently a position with a marketing communications agency. Carolyn dedicates this short story in loving memory of her mother Helen.

Elaine Morgan is an award winning poet and freelance writer. Her works have most recently appeared in *The Poet's Domain*, *Out of Line*, *Earth's Daughters*, *Sacred Journey Journal*, *National Association of Poetry Therapy*, among many other journals and periodicals. She has received awards from *ByLine Magazine* and The Poetry Society of Virginia. She is a three-time Senior Poet Laureate for the State of Virginia through the Kitchener Foundation.

Molly O'Dell, M.D., a practicing physician, Alegent Health Medical Director for Healthier Communities, and Adjunct Assistant Professor of Public Health and Pediatrics at the University of Nebraska Medical Center, has been a significant community health resource and advocate for over twenty years. In 1987 she became the Public Health Officer for a multi-locality public health district in the southern Appalachian Mountains for the Virginia Department of Health. Molly completed her MFA in poetry in July 2008 at University of Nebraska and has poems forthcoming in *Chest* and *JAMA*.

David W. Page, M.D., FACS is Professor of Surgery at Tufts University School of Medicine, Baystate Medical Center (BMC). He received an MFA in 2006 from the University of Southern Maine and has published numerous scientific papers, lay articles, three surgical textbook chapters and two reference books. *Body Trauma: A Writer's Guide to Wounds and Injuries* (Writer's Digest Books, 1996; second edition, Behler Publications, 2006) won an IPPY Silver Medal in 2007.

Diane Payne is the author of *Burning Tulips* and *A New Kind Of Music*. She has been published in hundreds of literary magazines. She teaches creative writing at University of Arkansas-Monticello.

Joel Peckham's essays, scholarly articles, and poetry have been published in numerous journals including *American Literature, The Black Warrior Review, The Literary Review, The North American Review, The Southern Review,* and *Under the Sun.* He is also the author of two books of poetry, *Nightwalking* (2001) and *The Heat of What Comes* (2008) with Pecan Grove Press. His chapbook, *Movers and Shakers* is forthcoming from Pudding House Press.

Joan Phillips, Ph.D., holds degrees in Interdisciplinary Studies, Art Therapy and Psychology and is faculty at the University of Oklahoma. She maintains a private practice of counseling/art therapy and sees a wide variety of clients. Her poetry has been featured several times in *Blood and thunder: musings on the art of medicine,* a literary journal published by the OU College of Medicine, is featured in *WordPictures: the poetry and art of art therapists* (2004), and in various literary journals.

Terry Sanville lives in San Luis Obispo, California with his artist-poet wife (his in-house editor) and one skinny cat (his in-house critic). He produces short stories, essays, poems, an occasional play, and novels. Since 2005, his short stories have been accepted by more than 120 literary and commercial journals, magazines, and anthologies. Terry is also a retired urban planner and an accomplished jazz and blues guitarist.

Paula Sergi is the author of the chapbook *Family Business* and co-editor of three anthologies: *Boomer Girls: Poems by Women from the Baby Boom Generation, Meditations on Hope,* and *A Call to Nursing.* The Wisconsin Academy of Sciences, Arts and Letters, along with the Hessen Literary Society, selected her as the 2005 cultural ambassador to Germany. A Wisconsin Arts Board Artist Fellowship recipient, her poetry is widely published, in such journals as *Rattle, The Bellevue Literary Review, Primavera, Crab Orchard Review,* and *Spoon River Poetry Review.*

Evelyn Sharenov is a writer and behavioral health nurse. She also holds degrees in literature, philosophy, and psychology. Her fiction and nonfiction has been published in numerous literary journals as well as anthologies. She has received an Oregon Literary Arts grant and is a member of the National Book Critics Circle. She is at work on a collection of essays, some published or forthcoming in noteworthy literary journals, including *The New York Times*.

Claudette Mork Sigg is a retired high school English teacher. Presently she is an Art, History, and Natural Science docent at the Oakland Museum of California. She has been published in numerous anthologies such as *Natural Bridge, Atlanta Review*, and *The Journal of the American Medical Association* as well as in *Love After 70* and *Illness & Grace/Terror & Transformation*.

Matthew B. Smith, M.D. is a gastroenterologist who has been in private practice in a suburb of Chicago for the last seventeen years. He has published original research articles in medical journals on topics ranging from Navajo Indian alcohol use to various topics in gastroenterology.

Robert P. Sticca, M.D., FACS graduated from the University of Connecticut School of Medicine and did his general surgery training at Boston University. He spent ten years as Associate Director of Surgical Education in the Greenville Hospital System in Greenville, South Carolina, and is currently Chairman of Surgery and the Director of Surgical Oncology at the University of North Dakota. This is his first creative nonfiction publication.

Maxine Susman's poems have appeared in several dozen journals and anthologies, including *Poet Lore, Paterson Literary Review, Alehouse, Dogwood Journal, Colere,* and *Blueline*. Her chapbooks are *Gogama* (2006), *Wartime Address* (2009), and *Familiar* (2009). Recent awards include an Allen Ginsberg Contest 2009 honorable mention. Professor of English at Caldwell College and member of the Cool Women performance group, she lives in Highland Park, NJ.

Sylvie Terespolski's writings have included magazine articles that appeared in *Insights* (McGill University), *Main Line Magazine, The English Journal*, op-eds in the *Philadelphia Inquirer*, and short stories in *Love after 70, Double Lives, Reinvention & Those We Leave Behind* and *The Reconstructionist*. She has works in perpetual progress that include three plays and an historical fiction novel titled *The Jew and the Pope*.

Timothy Francis Urban is a Writing and Literature major with a minor in Philosophy at Emmanuel College. He is highly influenced by existential writers in the same vein as Albert Camus and Milan Kundera. "The Sweet Life" reflects his interest in existential philosophy, and it is also his first published narrative.

Claudia Van Gerven teaches writing in Boulder, Colorado. Her poems have been published in a number of journals, including *Prairie Schooner* and *Calyx*, and in numerous anthologies. She has been nominated for the Pushcart Prize. Her chapbook, *The Ends of Sunbonnet Sue,* won the Angel Fish Press Poetry Prize and her full-length manuscript, *The Spirit String,* has been a finalist in three national contests.

Anne Webster's poetry collection *A History of Nursing* was a 2009 nominee for the National Book Award. She also contributed a chapter to *The Poetry of Nursing: Commentaries and Poems by Leading Nurse Poets*. Her poems have appeared in the *New York Quarterly,* the *Southern Poetry Review,* and *Intensive Care*. Her essays have been published in *Rattle, Final Moments, and A Call to Nursing*.

Gary Young's books include *Hands, The Dream of A Moral Life, Days, Braver Deeds*, and *No Other Life,* which won the William Carlos Williams Award. His most recent books are *Pleasure,* and *Bear Flag Republic: Prose Poems and Poetics from California.* Last year he received the Shelley Memorial Award from the Poetry Society of America. He teaches at the University of California, Santa Cruz.

GUEST EDITOR

PHYLLIS LANGTON, Ph.D., R.N., Professor Emerita, Sociology, George Washington University, is the author of more than 25 books and articles. She holds a doctorate from UCLA and an active registered nurse license from California for over 50 years. Her interest in creative non-fiction began in 2000 when her husband was diagnosed with Lou Gehrig's disease (ALS) and given six months to live. She received fellowships to write her memoir of this journey from Hambidge, Robert MacNamara Foundation, and the Ragdale Foundation. Three chapters from her memoir "Not Dead Yet: Living Well with Six Months to Live" have been published in anthologies, with the fourth in this anthology. She served four years as executive secretary of the DC/MD/VA ALS Board to educate the public and support families with ALS. She lives in McLean, Virginia.

EDITORS/PUBLISHERS

HEATHER TOSTESON holds an M.F.A. in Creative Writing (UNC-Greensboro), a Ph.D. in English and Creative Writing (Ohio University), and a Diploma in the Art of Spiritual Direction (San Francisco Theological Seminary). She has worked as a science writer and editor, executive editor of two public health journals at Harvard Medical School, and in health communications at the Centers for Disease Control, with a focus on communication across professional disciplines, racism, social trust, and how belief systems develop and change. She is the author of *The Sanctity of the Moment: Poems from Four Decades, Visible Signs, Hearts as Big as Fists,* and *God Speaks My Language, Can You?*

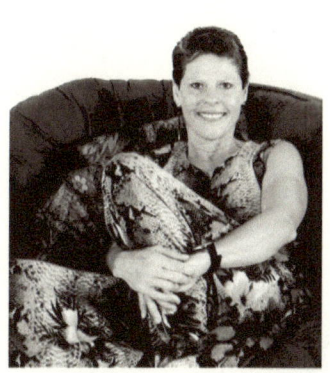 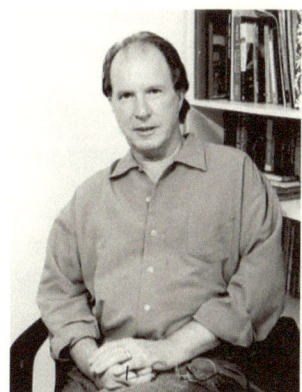

CHARLES BROCKETT, having worked from an early age in a small book bindery co-owned by his father, is enjoying his second career as a book publisher and co-director of Universal Table. He has written two well received books, *Political Movements and Violence in Central America* and *Land, Power, and Poverty: Agrarian Transformation and Political Conflict in Central America,* and numerous social science journal articles. A political science professor, he is a recipient of several Fulbright and National Endowment for the Humanities awards and has taught at Sewanee: The University of the South for thirty years. His Ph.D. is from UNC-Chapel Hill.

See our booklist and calls for submissions for new anthologies
www.universaltable.org
wisingup@universaltable.org

www.ingramcontent.com/pod-product-compliance
Lightning Source LLC
Chambersburg PA
CBHW030350020726
47493CB00003B/756